DEALING WITH FORCE

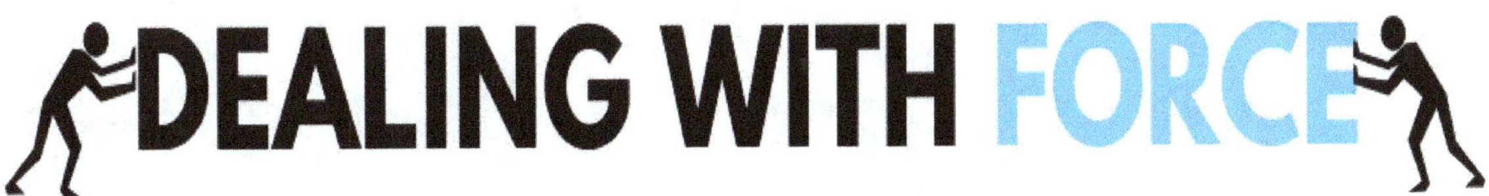

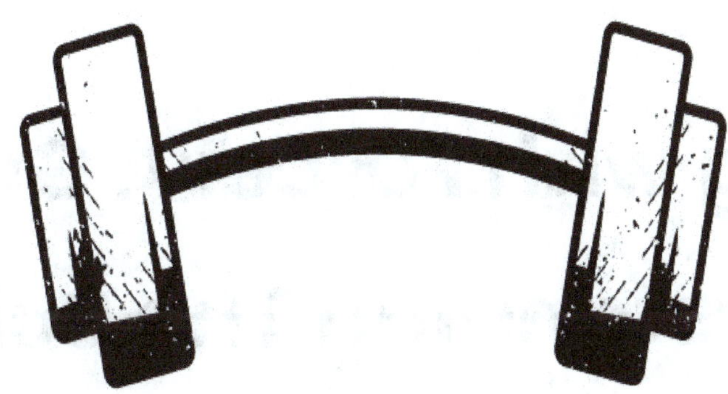

Understanding Simple Concepts to Master the Exercise Game

Tahran Gotla

Dealing with Force: A Guide To Understanding The Science Behind Exercise Mechanics

TABLE OF CONTENTS

PREFACE

I never thought I would take up physics again after I dropped it as a subject back in seventh grade. However, things have changed. From not wanting to take physics classes and read a physics text to writing an e-book on concepts revolving around forces and how forces affect us.

This e-book aims to provide a conceptual understanding of how forces interact with us, how forces are a part of our life, and how we interact with forces. By the end of this brief and thorough conceptual learning, you will be able to see what exercise truly is and determine with ease what works during an exercise. This e-book provides a solid base of physics and its implications when talking about exercise.

I hope this text gives you an edge over what you may already know. I hope you enjoy this one.

PREFACE

FUNDAMENTALS OF FORCE

I needed a thorough understanding of what **force** means to explain it without stuttering. I have now realized that simply **mugging up** definitions doesn't make it easier; rather, it minimizes the chance of **understanding and applying it** to work-related problems (exercise in this case).

To help understand the **concept of force**, let's start by covering the questions: "**WHAT** is Force, and **WHY** should you care about force"?

To get to the point:

In simple words, **Force** is "**a Push OR a Pull**."

That's as simple as it can get. A force is an action causing either a "**Pushing Movement**" or a "**Pulling Movement**."

Was it complicated?

No, right?

However, can you sense a "BUT" coming?

BUT...

The concept revolves around how a force **acts** upon an object, **impacts** an object, and **manipulates** an object and the subsequent **result** of the force. The **study of** Bio-mechanics is how we, as humans, **experience** forces, the **result** of forces, and how we **manage** these forces not only during exercise but also during daily living.

To make reading this definition easier, let's break down the words into two.

Bio: Pertaining to Biology/Human

Mechanics: The study of how forces act on something and the result of those forces. Although there are several different branches within the umbrella of "Mechanics," we shall be majorly covering "Rigid Body" Mechanics in this text.

Rigid means that objects in focus are considered to be solid and fixed without any deformation that could potentially occur. In the human body, we shall consider our bones as rigid structures articulated together to form joints.

Force = Mass x Acceleration

Simply put, the **amount of force** is a function of the **mass of an object** and the **rate** at which the object is made to **accelerate**. Acceleration is the **change in velocity over time**.

When understanding how forces impact us, we need to remember a few force characteristics:

1) Force has **magnitude**, measured in Newton.

2) Force has a **point of application**. For example, in a standing dumbbell bicep curl, the dumbbell applies a downward force on the palm.

3) Force has a **direction**. For example, as mentioned above, the dumbbell provides a "downward" force on the palm. Hint: The dumbbell has MASS, and that mass is **ACCELERATING** downwards due to **Gravity**.

These **three characteristics** make a **"force vector."** A force vector is a visual representation of the line of force that corresponds to force having **magnitude, direction, and point of application.**

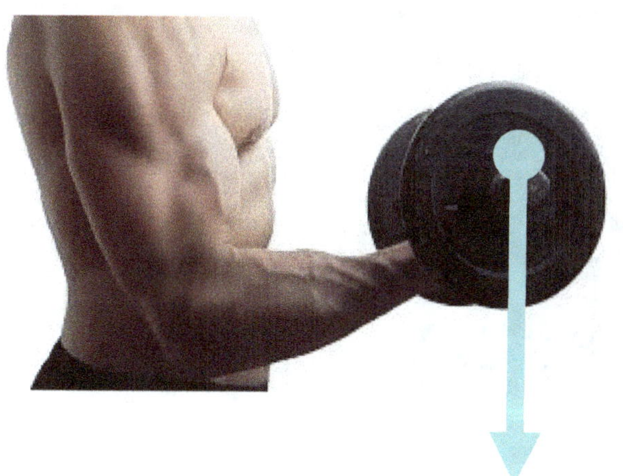
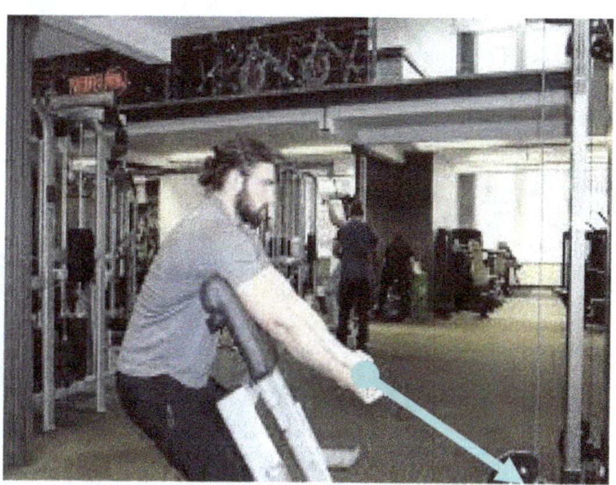

The arrowhead at the vector's end dictates the **force's direction.**

The length of the vector **dictates the magnitude** (Not calculated accurately in these pictures).

The solid dot at the beginning of the vector indicates the **forces point of application.**

When dealing with biomechanics, forces can be classified into two categories. The most basic classification of forces when dealing with the human body is

1) **External Force**

2) **Internal Force**

EXTERNAL *FORCE*

The above example showcases the amount, direction, and point of application of "external forces" on the body. These forces act on the body from external sources. There are multiple tools that we can use to experience such external forces. The above example showcases a Dumbbell and a Cable Machine.

In most instances, our body weight can be considered an external force. Body weight is the mass affected by the earth's gravitational pull on us.

In the following example, we can visualize Gravity's force vector.

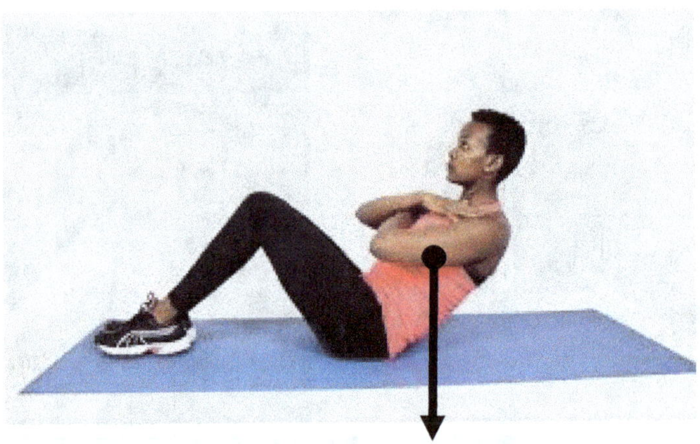

Mass vs. Weight

Does the dumbbell **"weigh"** 10 kg? Or is the "mass" of the dumbbell **10kgs?**

The **MASS** of the dumbbell is **10 kilos**. However, when taking 10 kilos and acceleration of Gravity into account, we get the **weight** of the dumbbell used.

10kgs x 9.8m^2 = 98N.

A deeper understanding of each type of external force will be covered later.

INTERNAL FORCE

Forces are produced within the body to **resist** the effects of **external forces**. Such forces are produced either **actively or passively** using our musculoskeletal system, which involves **skeletal muscles, connective tissues, and bony segments**. Internal forces can either cause **Motion, resist Motion, or limit Motion around a joint.**

Kinematics

The area of biomechanics involves **"motion."** In simpler words, this division of biomechanics revolves around describing Motion. Various variables are measured, such as **displacement, acceleration, and velocity of an object** in space, **without considering** the forces (push or pull) acting on that object. For instance, analyzing the bar path during a bench press or the distance traveled by the barbell during a barbell front squat.

Displacement of an object

The change in the position of an object is termed **displacement**. As simple as that. We shall cover two types of displacement, Translatory, and Rotary Displacement/Motion.

Translatory Motion

The Motion of an object in **one particular direction** (straight), wherein all points on a segment move **linearly**. This may only occur sometimes inside the body. This type of Motion may also be considered as "Non-Axial" Motion due to how it moves in space or glides through a given distance.

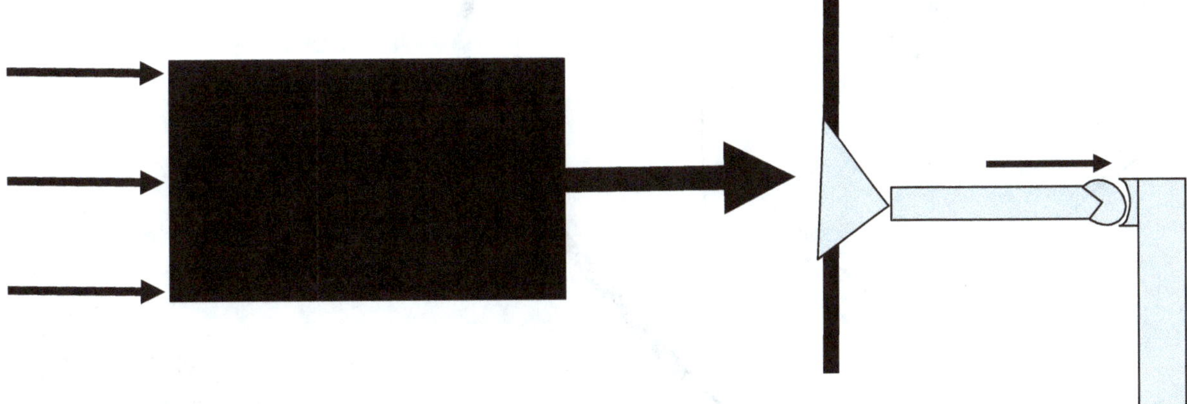

An Example of Translatory Motion in the human body

This is an example of pure translatory Motion. Imagine leaning against a wall using your palm. Here the wall exerts forces directly through your arm into the joint illustrated above.

During translatory Motion, every point on a segment moves a similar distance in a linear path without rotating around an axis.

Rotary Motion

The **Motion of an object around an axis of rotation** in a **curved pathway**. Like translatory Motion, rotary Motion does **not always occur in isolation** in the human body.

Notice that force is never "**curved.**" The result of **multiple linear force vectors** touching the circumference at a tangent creates **"rotation"** around an axis. Rotary motions can also be referred to as Axial Motion, in the sense that it is considered Motion around an axis and hence the term "axial."

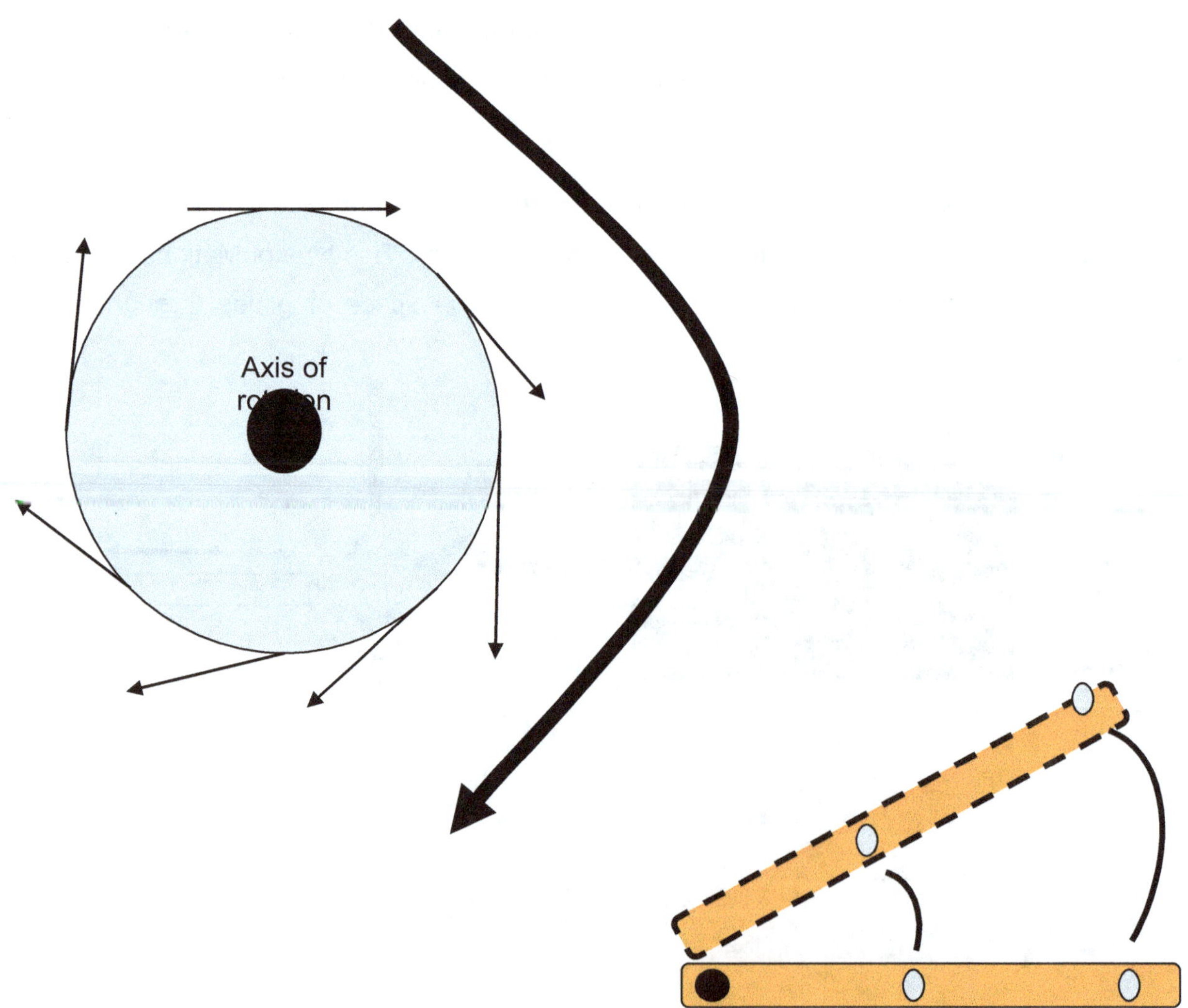

Another vital point to consider is that during any movement around an axis, a point closer to the axis will always move or be displaced to a lesser degree relative to a point further from a fixed axis.

This illustration exhibits the above, whereby the point closer to the axis moves through a smaller relative to the point further from the axis.

Curvilinear Motion (The amalgamation of the Translatory and Rotary Motion)

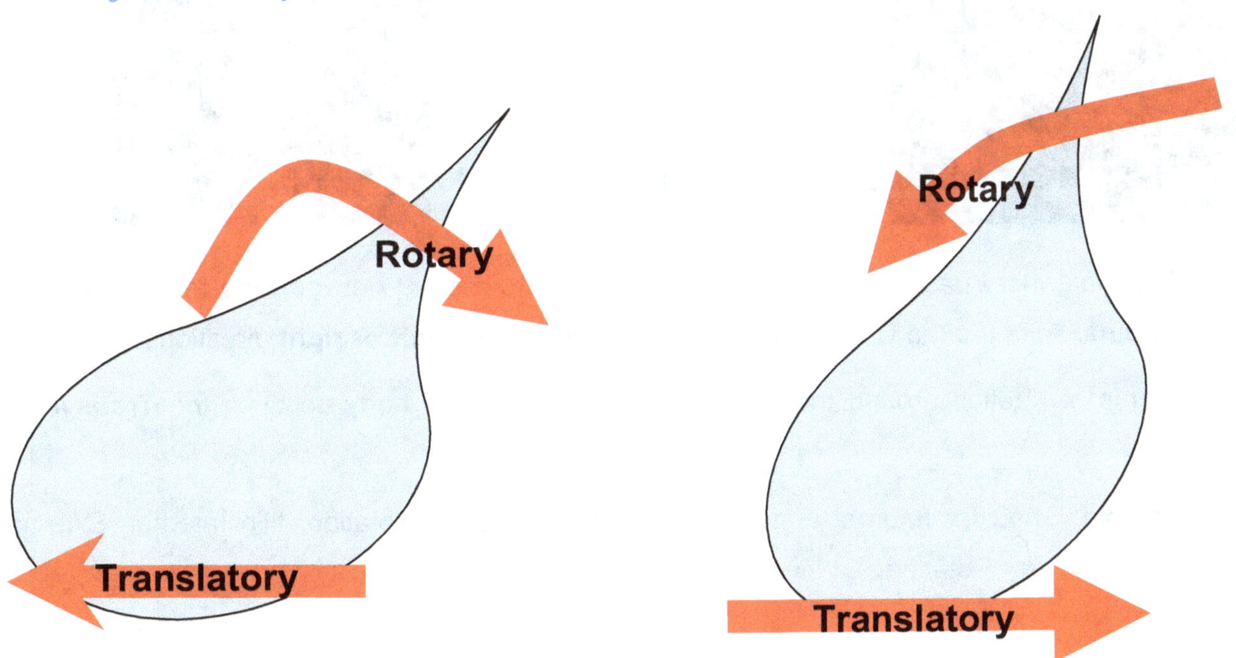

A make-shift representation of how there can be an integrated motion around a fixed segment.

Although the primary Motion here is considered as **"rotary"**, there will be subtle **forward translation** occurring as well during rotation.

As the upper segment rotates on the base of the rigid body, it is also moving forward.

Identifying where displacement occurs in the body around axes

Going back to mathematics, do you recall the **Cartesian Coordinate System**?

Do not worry; this isn't a math textbook; however, we will use the term **"axis"** here.

The Longitudinal Axis or the Vertical Axis

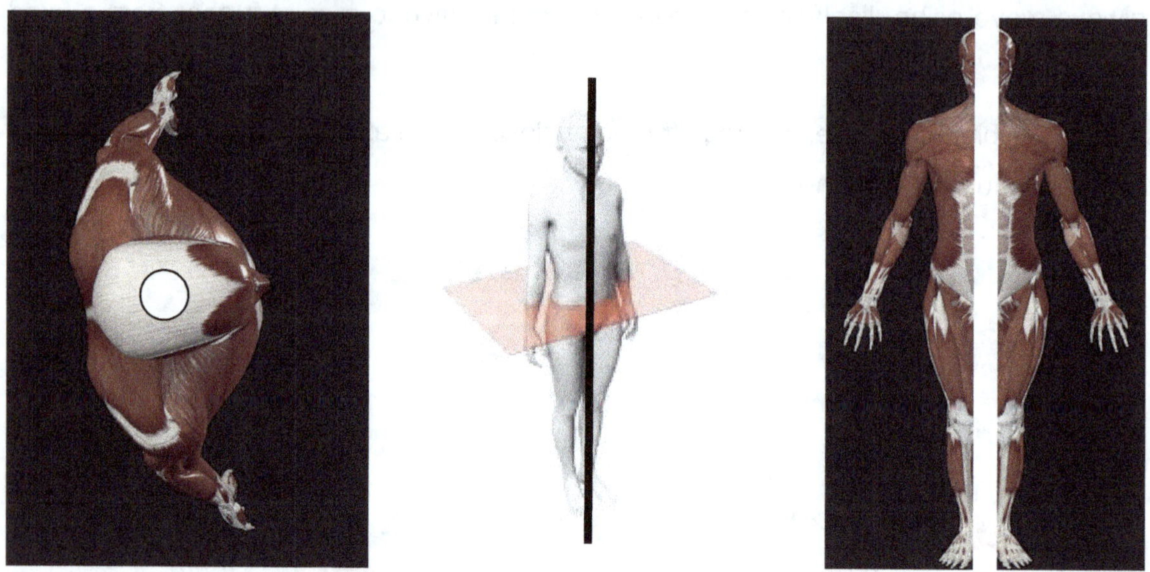

Visualize the "white" passing from the top of the skull to a point between the feet. This is the **Longitudinal Axis** around which the body can **rotate** in either **left or right** directions.

Movements of rotation around these axes of the joints in the body occur in the **Transverse Plane.**

For example, Shoulder Internal and External Rotation, Trunk Rotation, Hip Internal, External Rotation, and Neck Rotation.

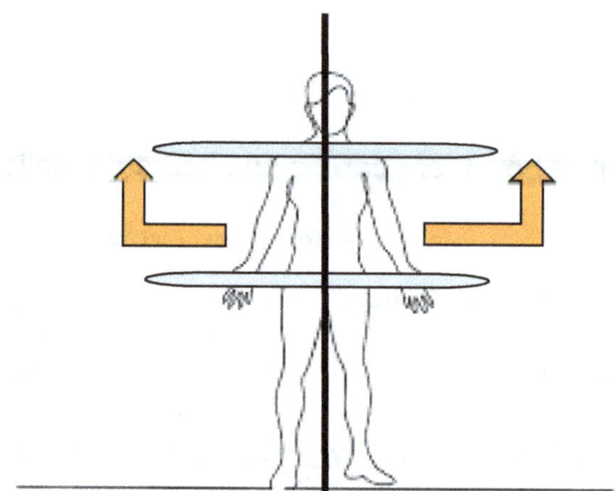

The illustration showcases rotation around a vertical/longitudinal axis, whereby the space between the two blocks highlights the transverse plane.

The Coronal Axis

An axis that runs side to side.

Visualize the white line passing through your joints from **left to right** or vice versa. This axis corresponds to a **rotation in the Sagittal Plane.**

For example, Shoulder Flexion and Extension, Hip Flexion and Extension, and Trunk Flexion and Extension.

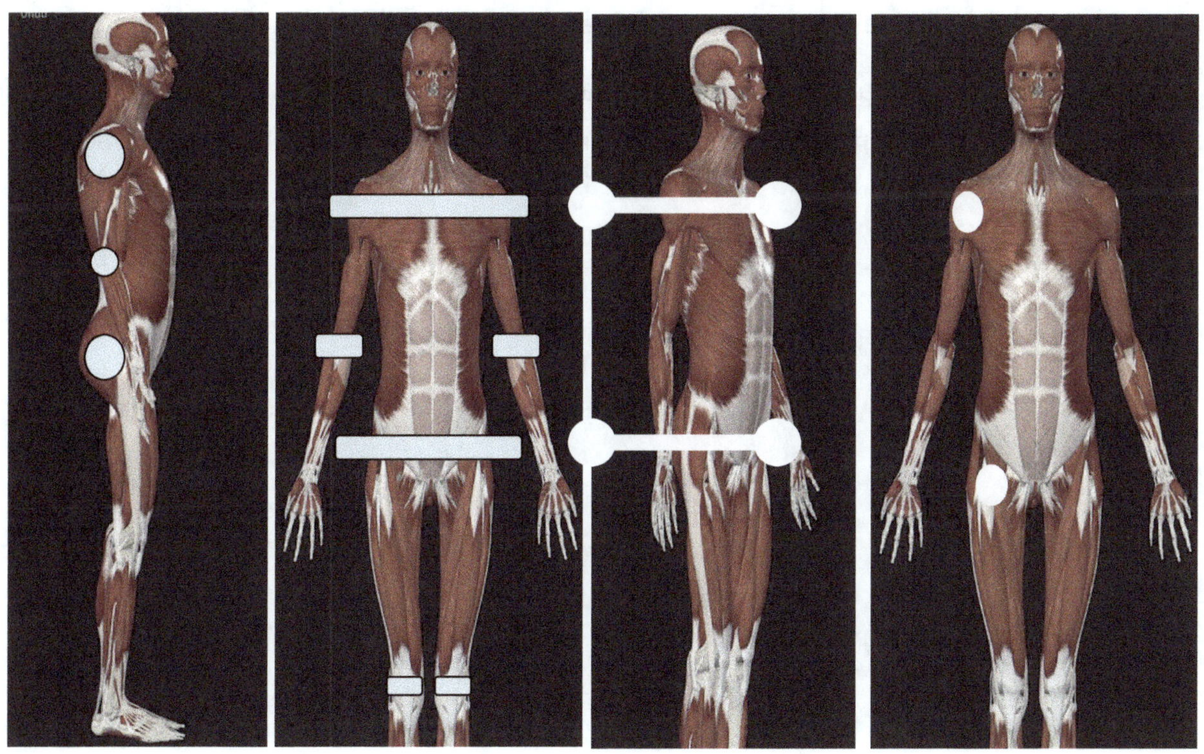

The Antero-posterior Axis

Visualize an axis running through a joint when viewing the body from the **front or back**. This allows your segments to rotate in the Frontal Plane.

For example, Shoulder ADDuction/ABduction, Hip ABduction/ADDuction, and Trunk Lateral Flexion.

Another point to make clear is that movement does not only occur around these fixed axes, but there could be **multiple permutations and combinations** around joints based on the degree of freedom a given joint provides to us, which provides us with an axis of rotation.

An example would be "lateral raises" in the scapular plane. This plane is not limited to moving around a rigid **Anterioposterior axis or the Coronal Axis** but lies somewhere in between.

UNDERSTANDING THE **RANGE** *OF MOTION*

Rotary Motion takes place around an axis of rotation.

The amount a segment can rotate around an axis is called **the Range of Motion** (ROM). ROM is typically measured in **degrees.**

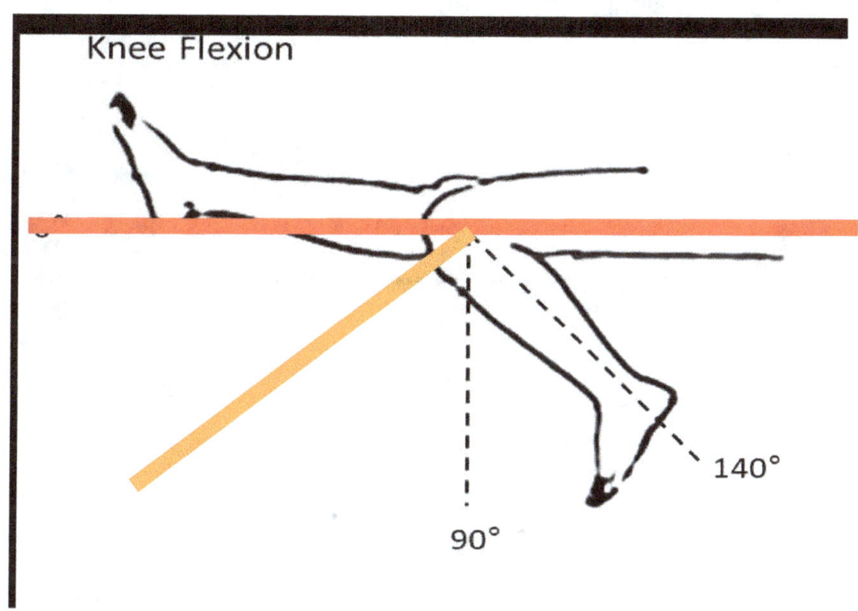

This is an example of a joint's range of Motion. An important point to take away from this illustration is that the angle of flexion or extension (around a coronal axis) will always depend on the relation between either limb segments and the line passing longitudinally through the knee joint.

Slightly flexing the knee creates 45 degrees of knee flexion. In this image, we see 90 degrees of knee flexion.' The red line constituents 0 degrees of knee flexion.

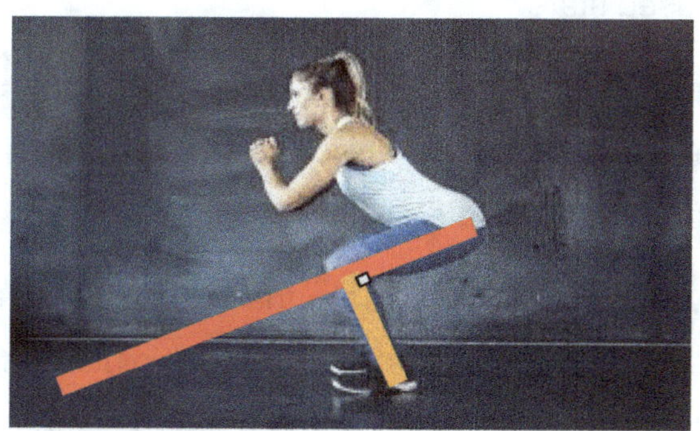

Understanding the relationship between the tibial and femur segments makes it easier to understand the angles of flexion/extension in this example. The amount of range available to a joint depends on various factors. A critical determinant of a joint's range of Motion is Joint Structure. A joint is a connection between two individual bony segments that are articulated together.

Certain joints in the body have articulating structures that allow a considerable range of Motion or limit the range of Motion to a significant degree.

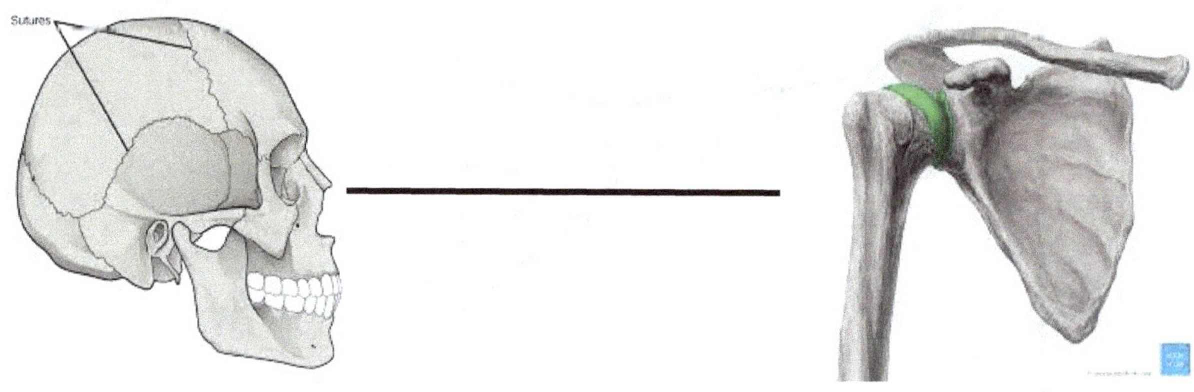

There lies a spectrum between which a joint lies in terms of structural limitations to Motion.

On the left side of the spectrum are joints that do not allow significant Motion. On another side of the spectrum are joints that are pretty mobile. Certain joints are considered "fused" joints where bony structures are tightly bonded to one another via connective tissues. There is less restraint relative to "fused" joints.

The factor differentiating the range of Motion is that the skull on the left has bones forming together as puzzle pieces in a fused state.

In contrast, the glenohumeral joint is an articulation between the humerus head that fits into a shallow socket called the Glenoid Fossa. The structure of the Glenohumeral joint allows a greater scope of movement relative to most joints.

When dealing with exercise, we rely more on joints that allow considerable movement. For instance, The Shoulder, Knee, Hip, Elbow, Wrist, and Ankle joints. Based on joint structure, features of bony segments that make up a joint, muscles that cross the joint, and ligaments and connective tissues that work around the joint are important determinants of the range available to the joints mentioned above.

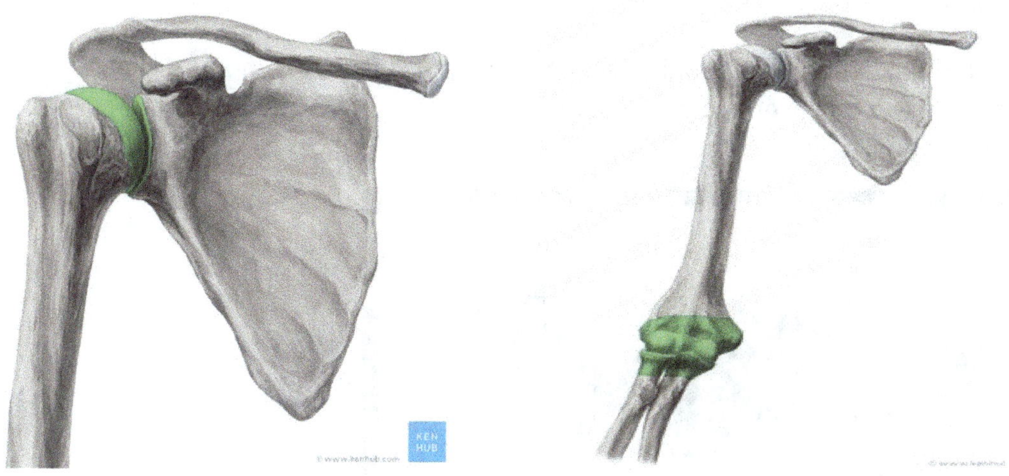

The above illustration showcases structural differences between the Glenohumeral and the Elbow Joint. Both joints differ from each other considerably in terms of articulating structures and movement pattern possibilities. The way the humeral head fits into the glenoid fossa (socket) varies relative to how the humeral end fits into the articulating surface of the Radius forearm bone.

Due to the Glenohumeral joint being a "ball and socket" joint, we see movement in multiple planes around different axes. However, in most instances, the elbow joint allows movement in only one plane around one axis.

Although the joint structure and its implications for exercise will be covered soon, we need to consider fundamental structural realities that can limit one's range of Motion.

The joint structure can set objective limitations for most. Still, inter-individual variations and within-individual differences have to be respected when dealing with various populations as an exercise professional.

LET US GET BACK TO FORCES FOR NOW

Let's recall three essential characteristics of a force vector:

A force vector has:

- A length that defines its magnitude. Let's look at another example:
- An arrowhead representing its direction
- A point of application.

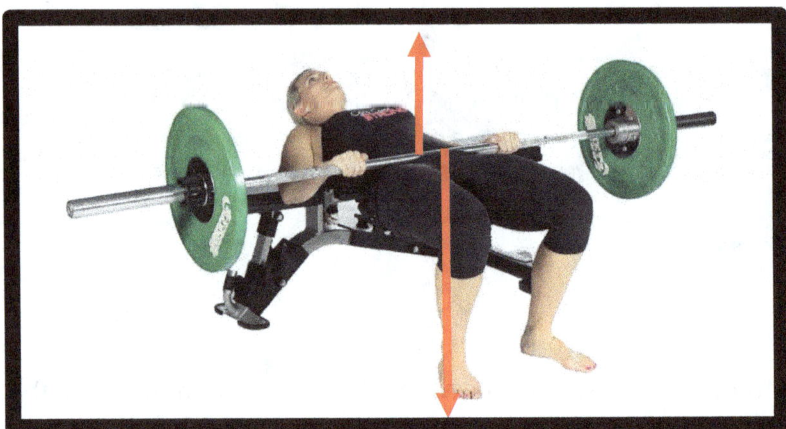

Here, we see two force vectors—one facing downwards towards the lady's torso and the other facing upwards towards the bar.

Since the force's magnitude is unknown, we shall not bother about the length of the vector. Instead, we need to consider its point of application and direction. This barbell only wants to move in one direction towards the pull of **Gravity** (downwards).

The barbell has **mass**, which is **accelerating** at 9.8m/s^2 **downwards**.

Speaking about gravitational forces leads us to understand the concepts revolving Center of Mass Or the Force of Gravity.

The force of Gravity is concentrated at an object's center of mass. More specifically, the force of Gravity acts at a specific point. This specific point is termed the Center of Gravity. The Center of mass refers to the point on an object/segment around which the entire mass of that object/segment is concentrated around. That particular point is called the "Center of Gravity."

Most objects have mass due to the matter it is made up of; objects have a center of mass.

Think of it this way.

Take a straight rod made of steel and try balancing the same on a fixed pivot. You will notice how the rod will only balance when you place the centermost point of the rod on a pivot.

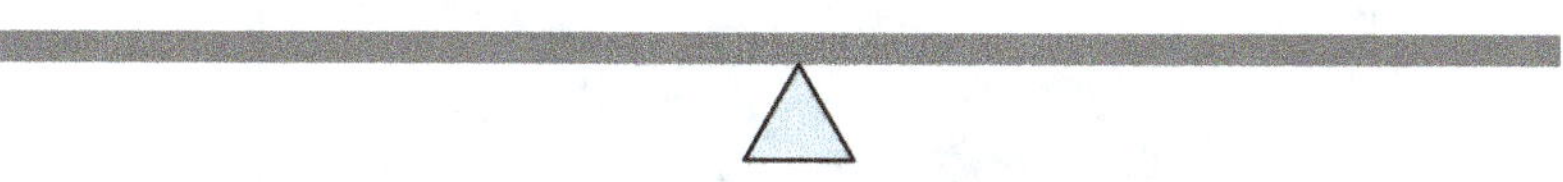

But what's the point of this illustration? There is no way that we as humans as such pristine symmetry.

That's a great thought!

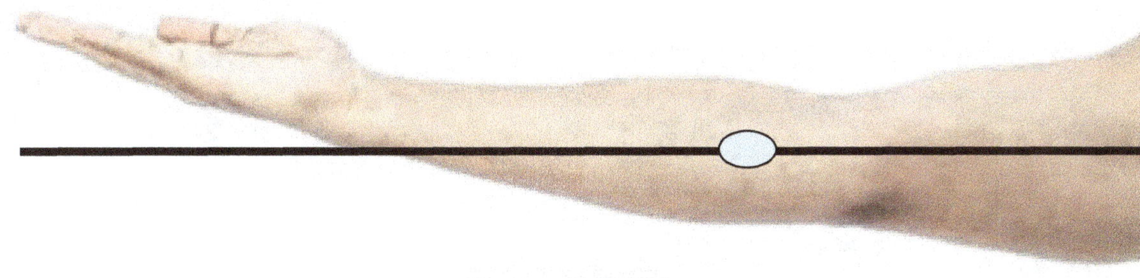

It gets slightly nuanced when dealing with human body segments.

The center of mass in this example is not in the center of the arm. When analyzing human body segments, we need to understand that because we are not symmetrical, we have mass distributed unevenly, which means the center of mass may not always be considered to be in the center of a given segment.

The upper arm (humerus) contains much more mass than the forearm. This shifts the center of mass towards the humerus.

Thus, as a rule, when a segment is not considered to have its mass distributed equally, we tend to have its center of mass closer to the heavier side.

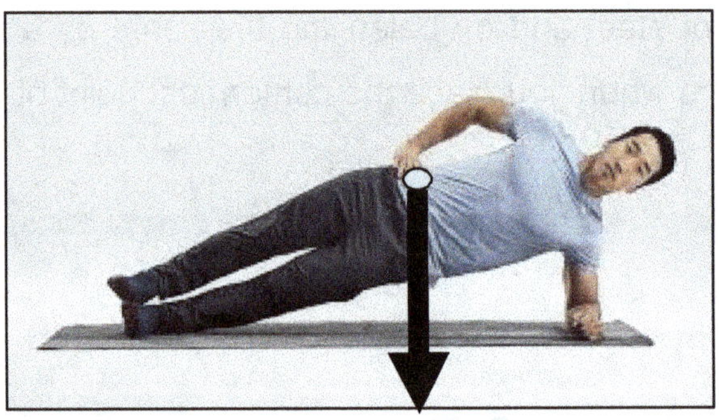

Example 2: The center of mass of this gentleman doing a side plank would be somewhere around the border of this pelvis. We need to consider that his left forearm is resting on the ground. That removes the forearm from the picture; hence, we do not consider that segment when analyzing the center of mass.

CONCEPTS REVOLVING AROUND <u>**COM**</u>

BALANCE AND STABILITY

The ability to maintain one's center of mass over one's base of support. The base of support refers to the area you have been placed over.

For instance, when standing on two feet, the base of the support consists of the area between the two feet. When seated on the chest press machine, the base of support is now the base of the machine, which contacts the floor.

There will always be **greater degrees of balance** when one manages to maintain their centre of mass over their base of support. The **larger** the base of support, the **greater** the **chance** of balancing oneself.

Moreover, the **closer** one COM to the ground, the **greater** the **chance** of balancing oneself.

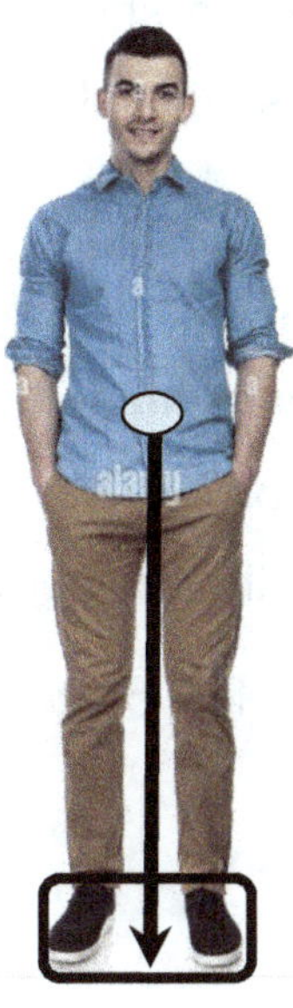

The **larger base of support** allows the individual to easily manage his center of mass within the area. This allows an improved ability to balance.

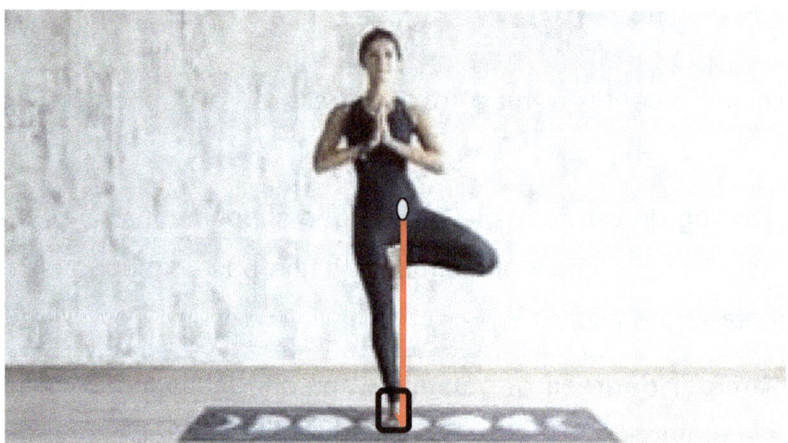

She has a reduced ability to balance due to a smaller base of support and having her centre of mass almost outside her base of support.

Stability refers to the ability of an object to show restraint toward forces affecting it. In other words, an object's capacity to return to its original position.

Factors that affect one's stability:

1) **The object's mass**
2) **The height** of an **object's center of mass** over the **base of support.**

In general, the greater the mass of an object, the more stable it would be relative to a lighter object, and the lower it's center of mass, the greater the stability.

Thus, an object with a lot of mass and a low center of mass within a large support base would be considered the most stable.

Coming back to the earlier example.

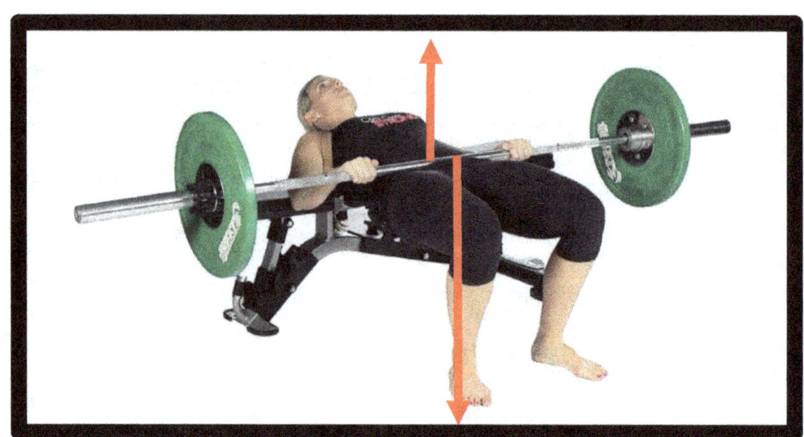

We now can understand why the barbell exerts a downward force at the center of the barbell. As long as the barbell is accurately loaded and the lady performing the movement is well-centered, the barbell's center of mass will always lie at the center. Gravity will act at this point downwards.

INTRODUCTION TO **KINETICS**

Forces can either **initiate Motion**, **stop** something from being in Motion, or **completely change** the direction in which an object is moving. Understanding these kinds of forces becomes important when analyzing exercises. The study of the forces that cause Motion is called **Kinetics**. Kinetics studies the forces that produce Motion—for instance, analyzing the forces in play during a barbell deadlift or understanding the amount of torque created by the hip flexors during a specific test.

In this chapter, we will be dealing with **External Forces** and **Internal Forces.**

What is the "**resistance**" in "**resistance training**"?

Is the resistance the dumbbell we hold during bicep curls? Is it the cables we pull towards ourselves during seated rows? Or Is it something that we cannot see but can experience?

Well, we definitely must take into account the aforementioned objects. But that only covers **50% of the resistance equation.**

50% of the equation, where **100%** equals **Torque**.

The load held in the palm during bicep curls tells us only a fraction of the story. The dumbbell has matter and, thus, has mass. This mass accelerates at $9.8 m/s^2$ in the direction of Gravity.

The result of this "external force" is Torque. Torque at the Elbow Joint.

Let us now ignore the influence of muscle force and think about what would occur at the elbow joint when a 10kg dumbbell is held.

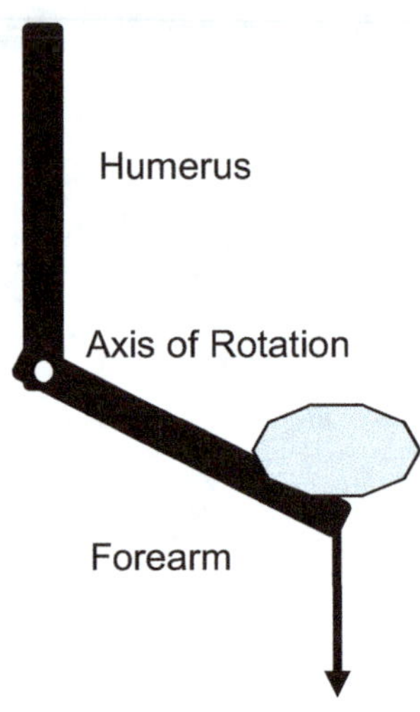

The angle between the humerus and the forearm increased. The dumbbell is producing elbow extension.

A better way of saying this would be the **dumbbell-produced elbow extension torque**.

The magnitude of torque produced depends on the load placed on the forearm and ALSO where the load is PLACED on the forearm.

Torque = **Force on segment** X **Placement of force on the segment**.

In more geeky words, Torque = Force X **Moment Arm**.

The **Moment Arm** is the other 50% of the equation.

The **Moment Arm** is simply the **"shortest" perpendicular distance** between the **line of force** and the **axis of rotation.**

Here we see how the load placed on the forearm acts at the elbow joint, which is 10 inches away.

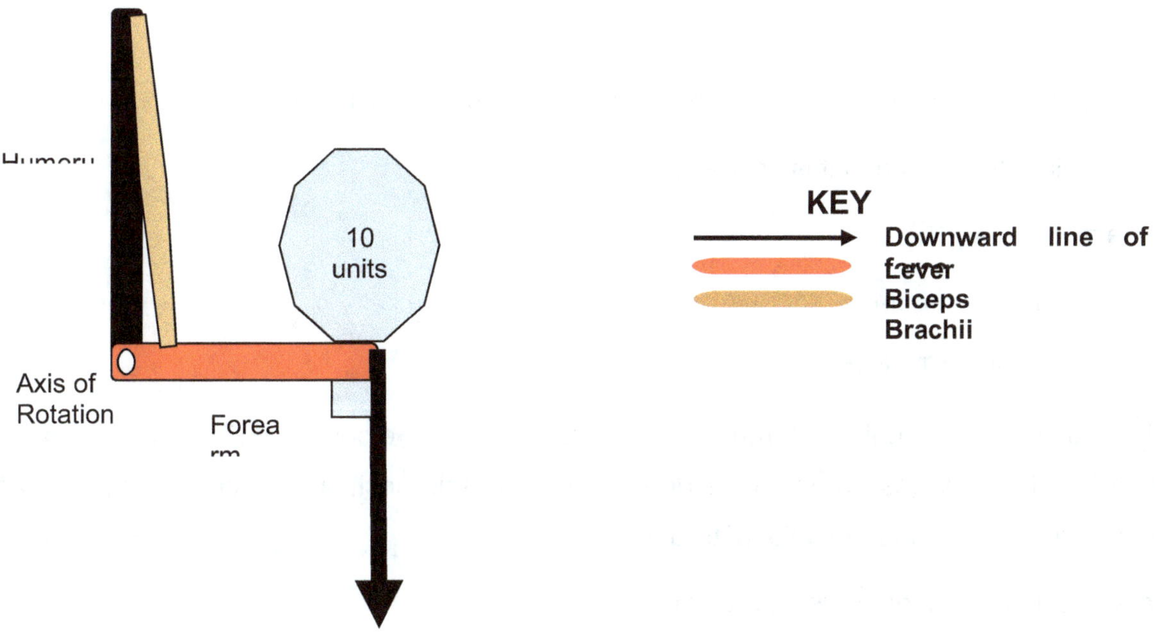

Torque = Force x Moment Arm

= 10 units x 10 units

= 100 units of Torque.

At this static point, 100 units of torque will be experienced. To maintain this position, the elbow flexors must work to create at least 100 units of torque.

Let's see what happens when we alter the joint position.

As the elbow goes into a more extended position, we see how the Moment Arm (in red) has reduced in length. The length of the forearm remains the same.

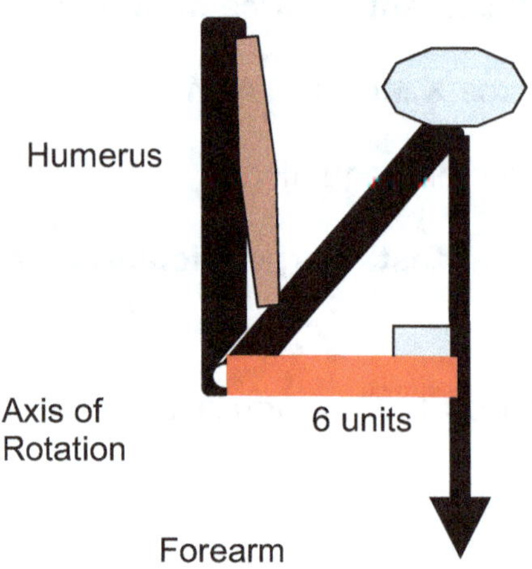

The forearm plays the role of a lever upon which the dumbbell acts downwards.

Let's calculate the torque in this scenario

Torque = Force X MA

      = ten units X 6 units

      = 60 units of Torque.

At this static point, 60 units of torque are experienced at the elbow joint. The amount of torque required by the muscles around the elbow to maintain this position reduces considerably from 100 units of torque to just 60 units of torque.

What does this say about muscular tension?

Since the torque requirements have reduced from 100 units to 60 units, the amount of tension (forces) produced by the elbow flexors reduces.

Let's cover the Hip Joint next.

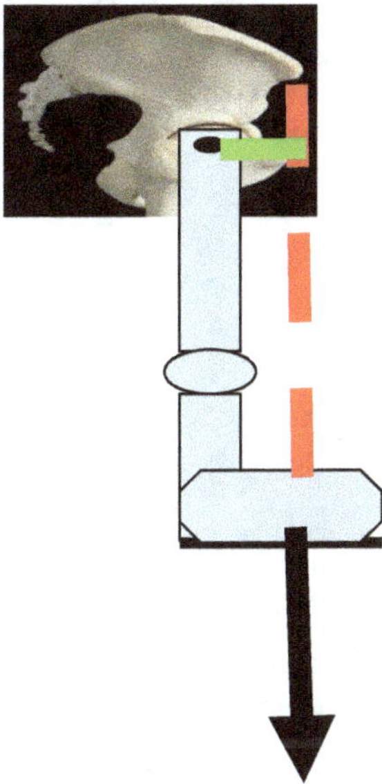

In this static image, the hip joint is extended with ten units of load placed on the foot. This load causes a force vector directly downwards in the line of Gravity. To figure out the relationship between the line of force and the joint's axis of rotation, we can extend the line of force using a dashed line upwards (Red dashed line).

This gives us a better understanding. It is easy to figure out the moment arm at the hip joint. At this position, we see a small moment arm which results in the hip extension torque at the hip joint.

The moment arm length comes out to be 2 inches.

Thus, we have ten units x 2 inches = 20-inch units of hip extension torque. Thus, the hip flexors must produce sufficient tension that causes at least 20-inch units of torque to offset the hip extension torque created by the dumbbell on foot.

As we use the hip flexors that cross the hip joint, we see the following changes in torque at the hip joint.

We now see, a longer moment arm as the hip went into flexion due to torque created by the Hip Flexors.

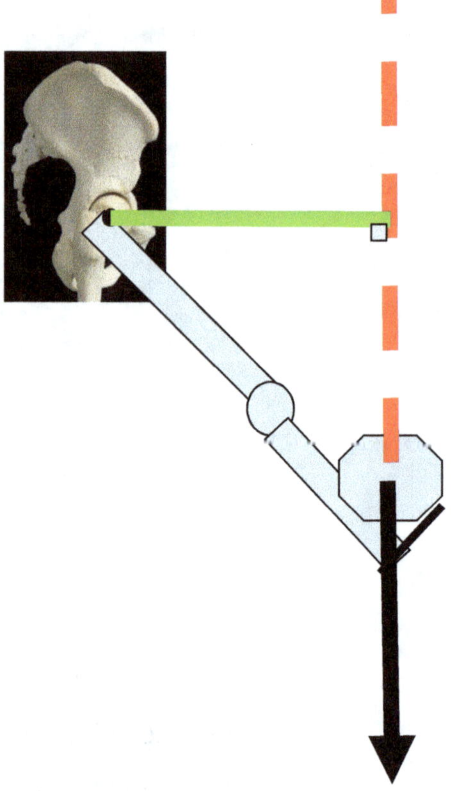

Although the dumbbell still provides ten units of force downwards, the amount of torque it produces at the hip joint had significantly increased relative to when the hip was in extension.

Torque = 10 units of force x 6 inches of Moment arm length

= 60-inch units of torque.

Thus, the amount of tension the muscles have to produce at the hip joint to oppose hip extension torque has increased dramatically.

From the above examples, we noticed that changes in the moment arm's length cause changes in the amount of torque experienced at an axis of rotation, specifically a joint.

MUSCLE **FORCES**

Skeletal muscle is a bundle of muscle fibers wrapped around in sheaths of connective tissues. Within a muscle belly, there are hundreds of bundles called Fascicles. Each of these fascicles contains muscle fibers or myofibrils. Each muscle fiber is also termed a muscle cell or Myo-cyte. Within each muscle fiber, numerous elements are named organelles, just like we see in other cells of the body. In particular, we are thoroughly interested in organelles called sarcomeres. Sarcomeres contain two vital protein filaments that are responsible for muscular contractions. When the muscle fiber receives its signal from the nervous system, it fires, resulting in a muscular contraction.

Simply put, electric energy gets converted into chemical energy to produce mechanical energy leading to movement or the restriction of movement.

The whole purpose of contracting is to create muscular forces called muscular tension. The tension produced could either be produced actively or passively.

Active tension is the tension produced via the interaction of the aforementioned protein filaments within the sarcomere of a muscle fiber. Passive tension is the tension produced via passive or non - contractile protein structures other than contractile protein filaments in the sarcomere. This tension is produced as the muscle fiber stretches or lengthens against the resistance caused by external forces. One of the main contributors to passive tension generation is a protein called Titin.

So why do muscles produce tension?

The most straightforward answer is to produce or restrict motion depending on what is demanded in a given scenario. More importantly, to produce torque, to oppose the torque caused by an external force.

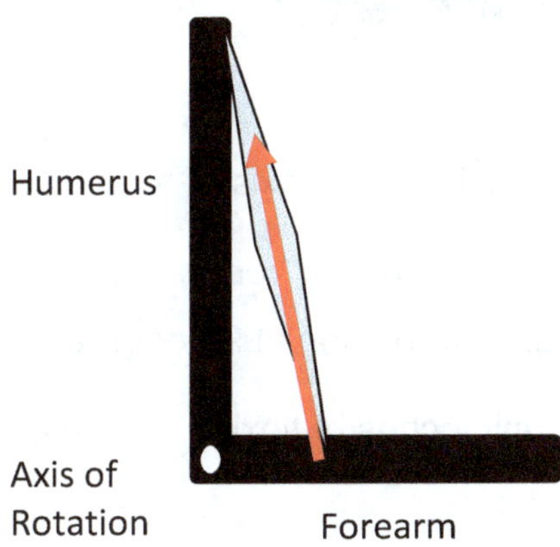

A force vector also denotes muscle force with magnitude, direction, and a point of application.

This figure showcases the force vector of the Biceps Brachi, one of the significant elbow flexors.

The Biceps attach on two bony segments. When required to contract, moving the "lighter segment" toward the heavier segment produces tension.

The radius, a bone that comprises the forearm, is one of the attachment points of the Biceps. We see a force vector running upwards at an angle from the biceps attachment point on the forearm. This is referred to as the "line of pull."

Internal Torque Production

In response to external forces creating torque at a joint, muscles produce their forces to counter the resistance (torque). This creates internal torque.

Internal Torque = Muscle Force X Length of Moment Arm.

INTERNAL MOMENT ARM

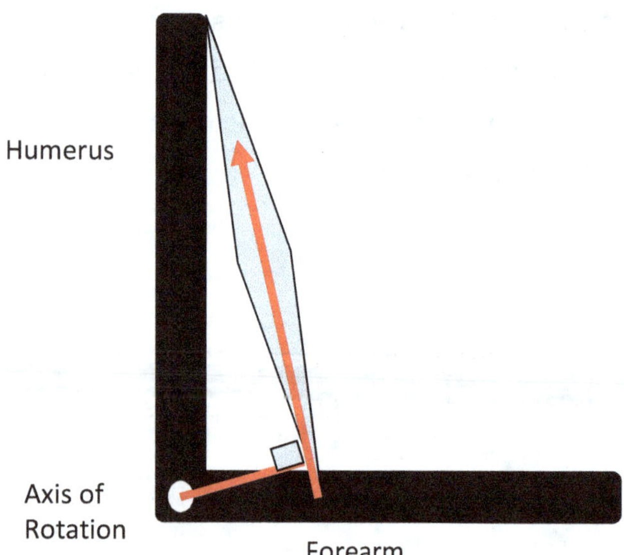

The perpendicular distance between the joint's axis of rotation and the muscle's line of pull.

Suppose the Biceps is producing 8 units of force, and the length of the moment arm is approximately 2 inches from the axis of rotation at 90 degrees.

Torque: 8 units X 2 inches = 16 unit inches of flexion torque at the elbow joint.

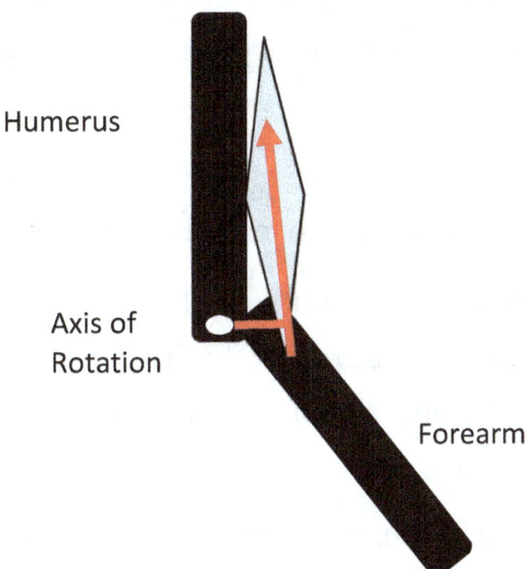

Look what happens as the elbow joint starts to extend. We see a reduction in the moment arm between the biceps line of pull and the joint's axis of rotation.

This occurs because the biceps line of pull creeps closer to the joint axis.

Let's assume that the bicep creates similar tension at this position.

The amount of torque produced here would be

= 8 units X 1 inch

= 4 unit inches of flexion torque at the elbow joint

But where is the resistance?

What are the biceps overcoming? There needs to be a reason for the biceps to produce sufficient tension to create elbow flexion torque in the counter-clockwise direction.

That reason elbow extension torque is produced by an external force acting on the forearm, a lever.

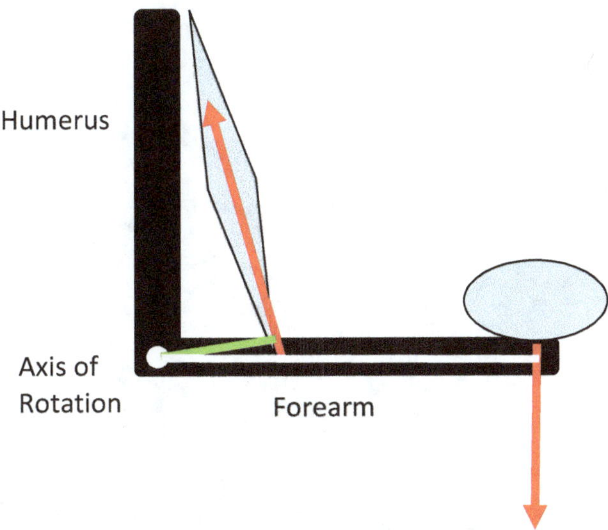

In this example, we see an integration of two forces acting at the elbow joint. An external force is represented by a dumbbell held over a person's palm, and the biceps line of action represents an internal force.

The amount of force the bicep needs to produce at differing angles of the elbow joint will depend upon the amount of torque it needs to resist due to an external force.

Let's create an interesting scenario: Suppose the load placed on the forearm is 10 units. And this load is placed 15 inches from the elbow joint. In this scenario, the perpendicular distance between the elbow axis of rotation and the line of force acting downwards is 15 inches—the length of the lever or the forearm itself.

The amount of torque this dumbbell produces at the elbow is the resistance the biceps have to overcome.

Elbow Extension Torque: 10 units x 15 inches

: 150 unit inches of Torque.

Suppose the biceps line of pull is approximately 2 inches from the joint's axis of rotation.

The amount of torque that the bicep needs to overcome, to keep the forearm parallel to the floor is 150 unit inches of Torque.

So, if the biceps line of pull is 2 inches away, it needs to produce at least 150 unit inches of torque at the elbow joint; this is the equation we need to complete.

The torque needed: Force of biceps X Moment Arm

150 unit inches: "x" X 2 inches

X = 75 units of force.

The force experienced by the dumbbell sitting on the forearm is countered by force produced by the biceps because elbow extension torque is checked by elbow flexion torque. Thus, when the biceps produce 75 units of force, the forearm remains parallel to the ground. We call this a state of equilibrium.

Elbow extension torque = Created by Dumbbell

Elbow Flexion torque = Created by Bicep

What happens when the biceps can produce a lot more tension?

Let's say the biceps produce 90 units of force, 2 inches from the elbow's axis of rotation. This would create more elbow flexion torque. The new torque created equals 180 unit inches of elbow flexion torque.

180 > 150.

This leads to elbow flexion; the biceps can be considered the winners of the fight.

Net torque = 30 unit inches in favor of the biceps.

Coming back to the example of you having your forearm parallel to the ground,

You are feeling lazy and may want to avoid creating greater bicep force.

The force you produce becomes 60 units of muscle force, placed 2 inches from the joint's axis of rotation.

This leads to an elbow flexion torque of just 120 unit inches, whereas the elbow extension torque to overcome remains at 150 unit inches.

This creates a net torque of -30 unit inches in favor of the external load placed on the forearm.

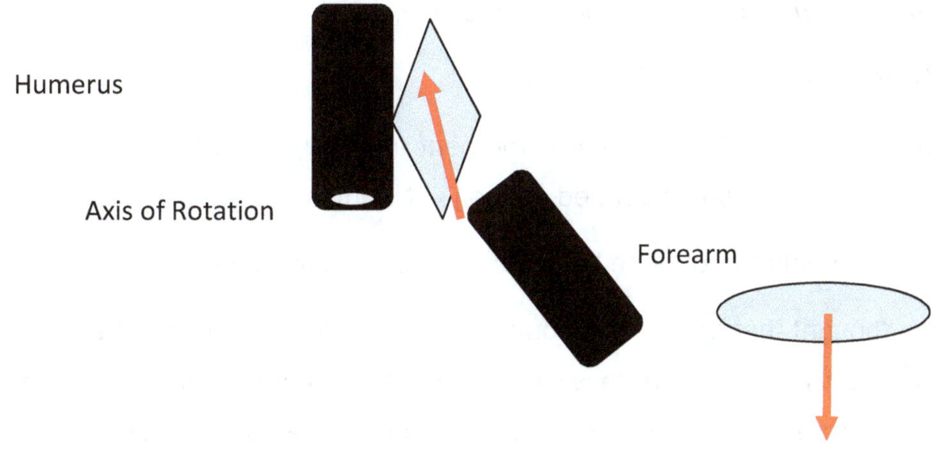

The result is **elbow extension.**

Things have changed.

The dumbbell providing ten units of external force remains the same. However, what happens to the torque produced at the elbow joint changes drastically.

The moment the arm between the joint's axis of rotation and the line of action passing through the dumbbell shortens as the arm is brought into slight extension.

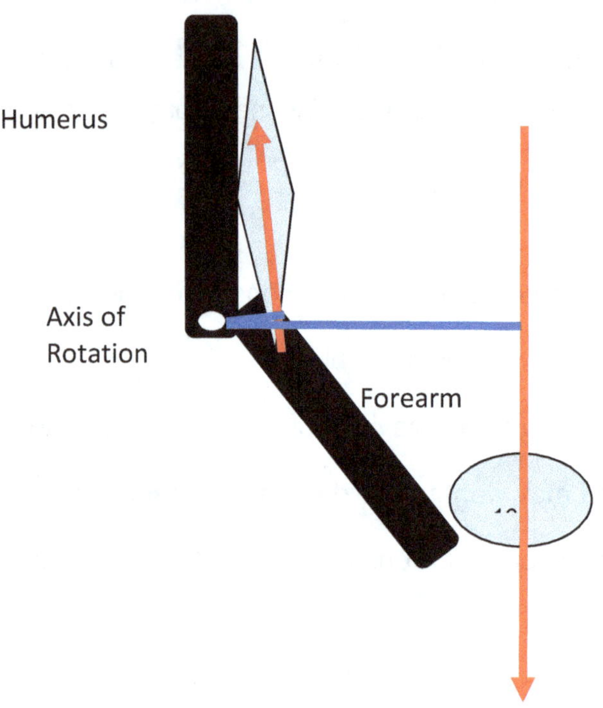

Torque experienced: 10 units X 8 inches

80 unit inches of elbow extension torque at the elbow.

Well, things have changed internally as well.

Look at the biceps line of pull. The internal moment arm between the biceps line of pull and the joint's axis of rotation has also decreased as the joint went into slight extension.

That means the amount of torque the biceps can produce diminishes.

You may have thought that the biceps would have a greater advantage due to the reduction in external torque. But that isn't the case! The amount of torque needed to offset the external elbow extension torque = 80 unit inches, and the force required by the biceps equals…

The amount of elbow flexion torque = Force of the biceps X MA

80 unit inches = "x" X 1-inch

The amount of force required by the biceps to maintain this position = 80 unit inches of elbow flexion torque.

Suppose there's confusion as of now based on what has been covered. I urge you to think of these numbers as simple proportions. For instance, think of it like this.

The amount of muscle force the biceps had to produce in the original example was 75 units of force. The moment the elbow went into extension, the amount of force the bicep required to produce increased to 80 units.

This occurred although the external torque at the elbow decreased to 80 from 150 unit inches.

Why?

Due to the reduction in the distance between the biceps line of pull and the elbows axis of rotation.

Only when the biceps produce 80 units of force will it match the external torque of 80 unit inches. Because 80 units of force X 1-inch moment arm = 80 unit inches of elbow flexion torque.

Please Note

This example isolates the biceps and the dumbbell placed on the forearm. In most scenarios, we have more than just the biceps producing elbow flexion torque; we can do more than just the dumbbell creating external forces. This changes the dynamic and the relationships that we have explored. Moreover, there are some musculoskeletal realities that we need to take into account, such as Muscle Length-Tension Relationship, Joint Forces, Inertial properties, Strength profiles, and so on.

But that is fine because this chapter's primary goal is to make it easier to understand complex situations later on.

UNDERSTANDING *FORCE ANGLES*

A force angle is formed between a force vector and its intersecting segment, which can be considered a "lever." A simple lever differs from a "lever arm."

A lever is a segment meant to rotate around an axis of rotation.

The distance between the axis of rotation and the point of application of a force vector makes a "lever arm."

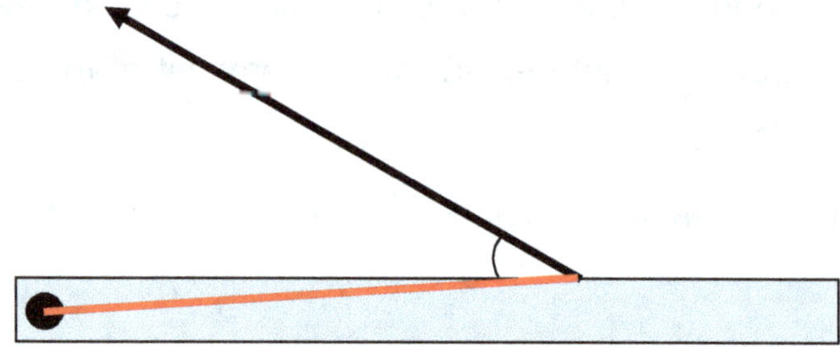

The solid red line denotes the "Lever Arm." This line connects the rotation axis to the force line at its point of application. The lever is the segment on which the force acts. Moreover, the force angle between the "lever arm and the force vector can be seen.

Force angles are essential because it tells us more about the length of the moment arm acting at a given axis of rotation.

Let's look at a simple segment with an axis of rotation and a force applied.

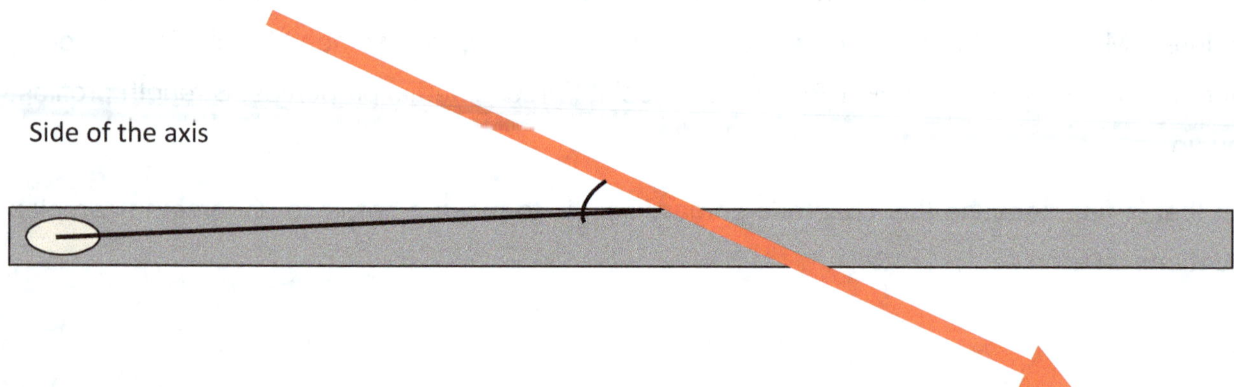

The angle formed between the intersection of the black segment and the force vector (Red vector) is the force angle.

Notice how the force angle is always measured on the side of the axis of rotation.

The moment arm between the line of force and the axis of rotation is as follows.

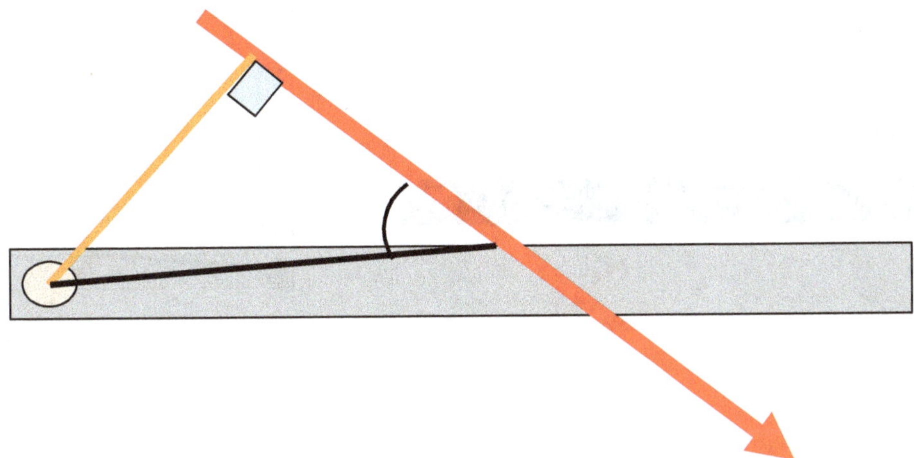

Let's explore what happens as we increase the angle at which the force vector intersects the segment.

1) **A 0-degree Force Angle** = No moment arm as the line of force passes directly through the axis of rotation. This force has no torque-producing capabilities.

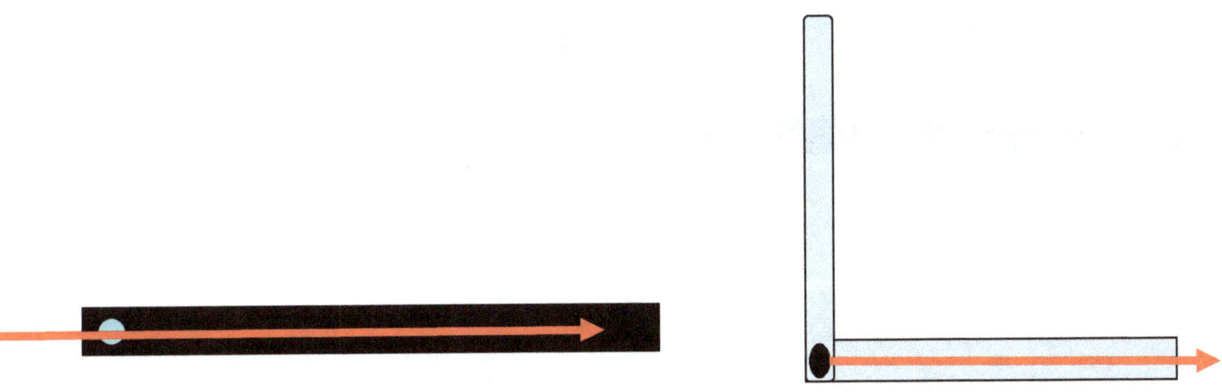

2) **A 30-degree Force Angle** = A moment arm is seen as the line of force passes at an angle through the segment.

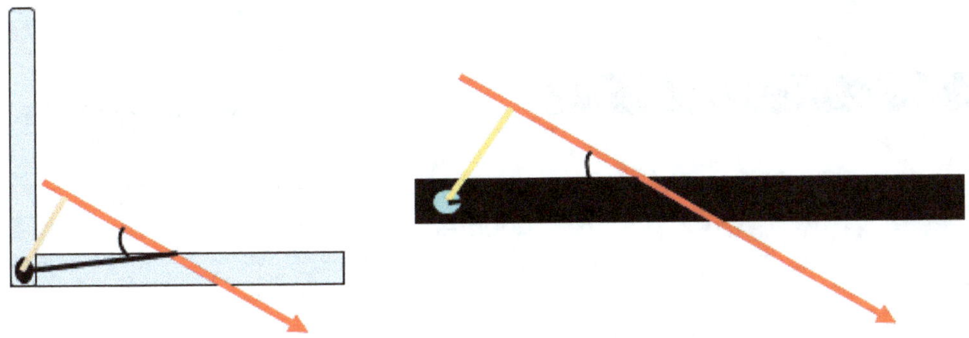

3) **A 45-degree Force Angle** = A relatively longer moment arm due to increased force angle.

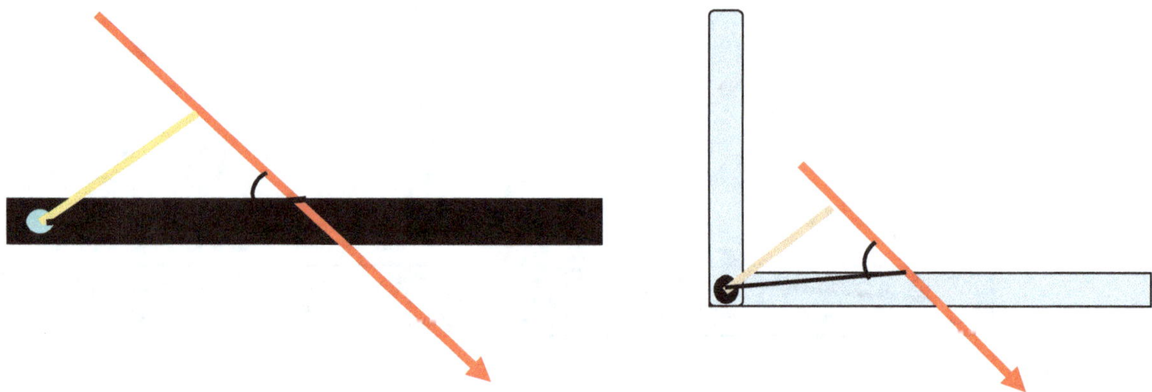

4) **A 90-degree Force Angle** = The longest moment arm due to a 90-degree joint angle to the segment.

5) A 135 - degree Force Angle = Smaller moment arm due to an increased force angle in the side opposite to the axis of rotation.

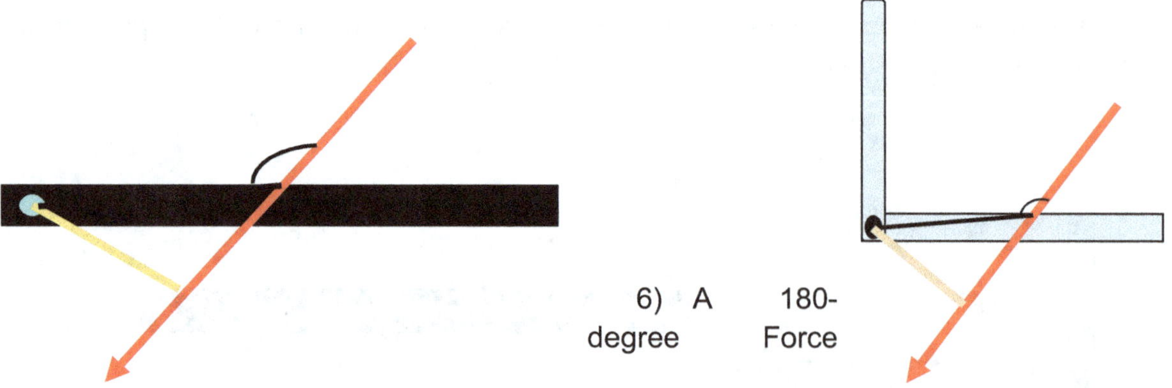

6) A   180-degree   Force

Angle = No moment arm due to the line of force once again passing through the axis of rotation.

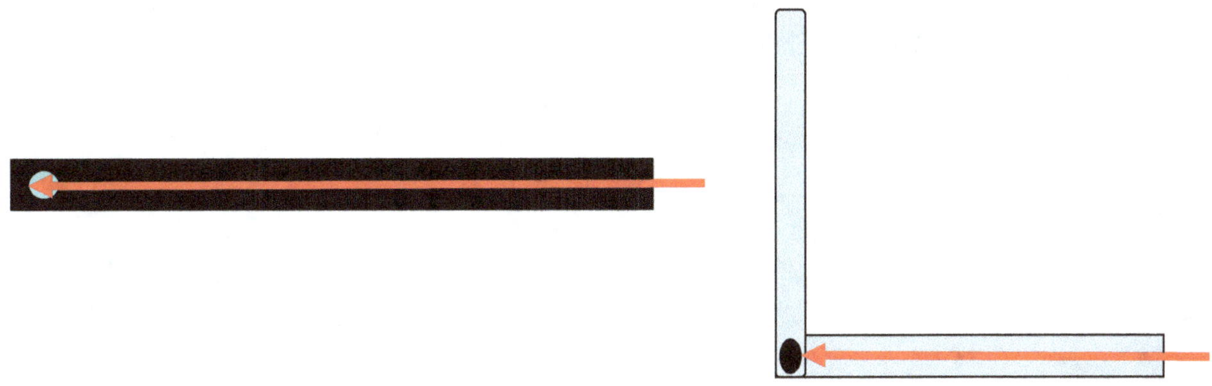

From these illustrations, we must consider **two** important implications:

1) When the line of force passes through the axis of rotation, NO moment arm is possible. Thus if there is no rotation around the axis of rotation, however, this force is not considered "ineffective." Although it is "ineffective" at producing rotary motion, it does provide other benefits. In the first illustration, the force tries to pull the lever apart from the axis. In illustration number 6), the force line pushes the lever into the axis of rotation.
2) When the line of force is at 90 degrees to the lever arm, the amount of rotation that force can cause is the most relative to other force angles. This is due to the largest moment arm between the line of force and the axis of rotation. This means the force shown in illustration 4) can produce the most rotation. But may need to be capable of having translatory effects.

Therefore, as the force angle goes from 1 degree to 89 degrees, the moment arm increases gradually until it is the longest at 90 degrees. And as the force angle goes from 91 to 179 degrees, its moment arm again decreases in length.

Let's take a look at real-life objects to get a crisper understanding of force angles.

This is a Landmine Row set up

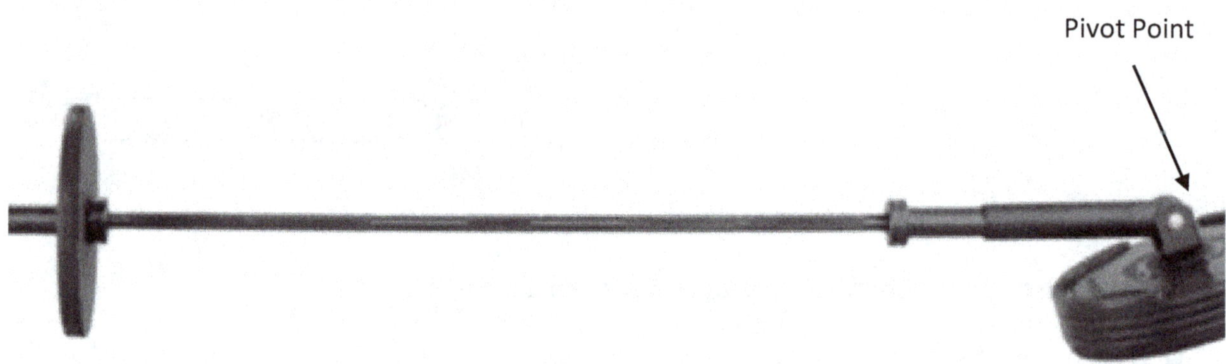

Let's find out the most efficient way to pull the bar to create rotary Motion around the pivot point (axis of rotation).

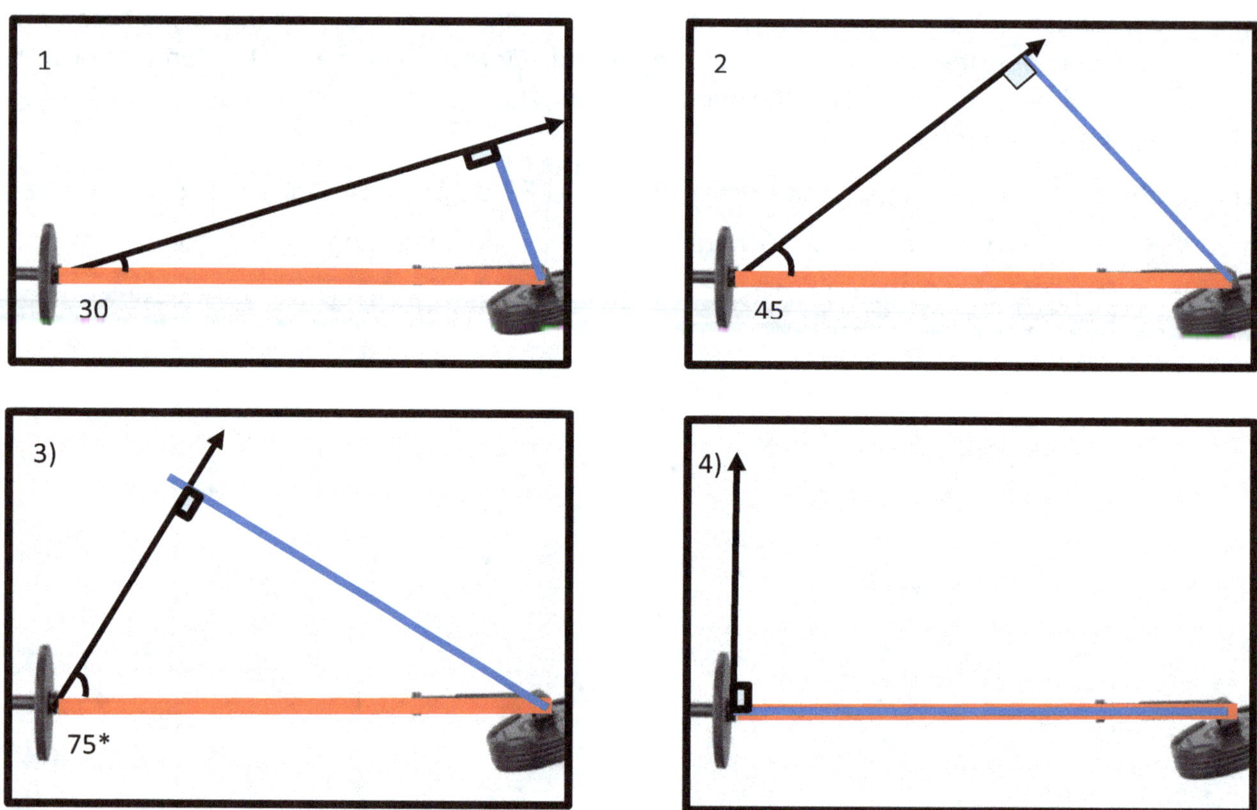

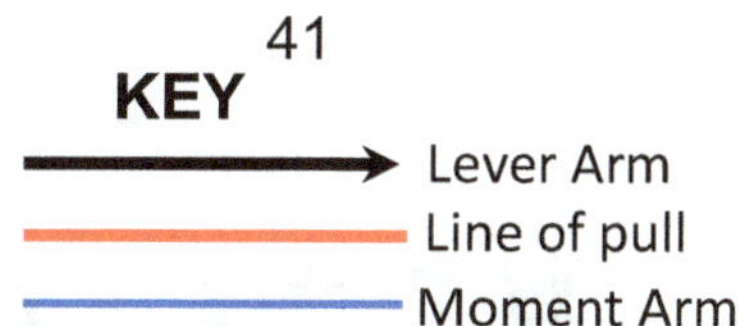

Illustration 1 showcases a force angle of 30 degrees between the line of force and the lever arm. In this situation, the external moment arm is the shortest, which does not create the most "rotary" effect at the landmine's pivot point.

However, as the force angle increases from 30 to 75 degrees in illustration 3, the length of the external moment arm increases. All less being constant, a longer external moment arm in illustration 3 would lead to a greater degree of rotary effect around the landmine's pivot point.

Illustration 4 showcases a longer moment arm due to a 90-degree force angle acting on the lever arm. This line of force exerted on the barbell would cause the greatest degree of rotation around the pivot point of the landmine setup.

For instance, imagine pulling on the barbell using a rope or using your arms at a 90-degree angle. All less being equal, you will be stronger relative to pulling at different angles on the same barbell and at the same point.

How does this apply to the human body?

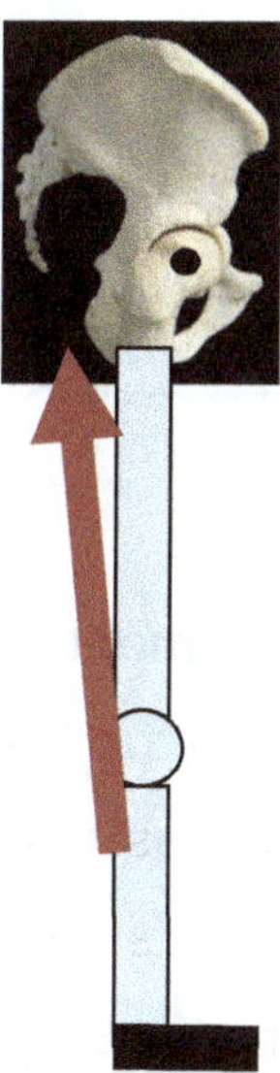

This illustration showcases the line of pull produced by the Hamstring Group of muscles. Three out of the four heads of the Hamstrings cross the hip joint and the knee joint.

One of the Hamstring's primary functions is to produce a force that results in knee flexion torque, mainly to oppose knee extension torque produced by external forces.

Given the above description, let's see in what part of the range of Motion, do the Hamstrings have a better advantage to cause rotation around the knee joint.

Please Note: The knee joint is the axis of rotation in this illustration. For simplicity's sake, we assume that the center of rotation remains constant and does not change as the joint continues to flex.

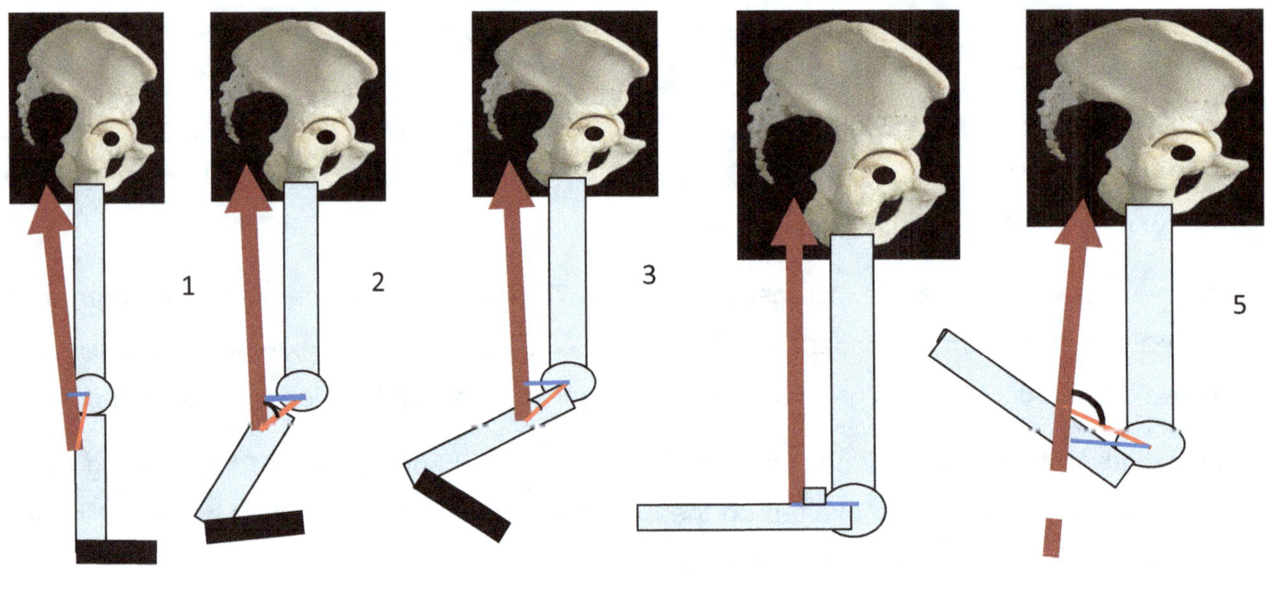

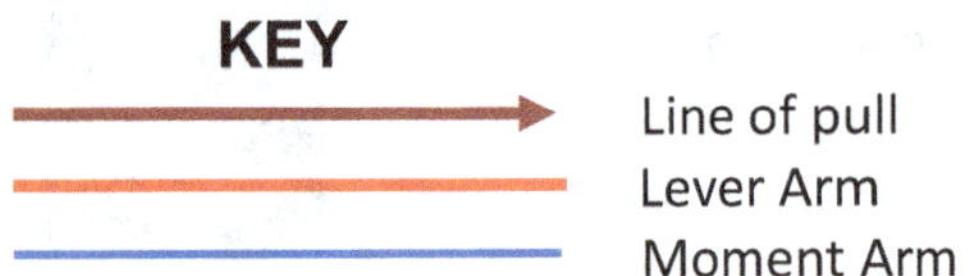

The moment the lower segment becomes parallel to the floor, we see a 90-degree angle between the Hamstrings line of pull and the lever (segment) on which it acts. At this position, the hamstrings have a favorable line of pull to cause the most amount of rotation around the knee joint's axis of rotation. This mainly occurs due to an increased internal moment arm that maximizes torque production to cause rotation.

In illustration 1) although we see a small moment arm due to a small force angle, the amount of rotation caused is minimal.

Moreover, as the knee flexed further, we see in illustration 5) that the moment arm tends to reduce as the force angle starts going over 90 degrees.

<u>UNDERSTANDING</u> *COMPONENTS OF FORCES*

In the previous section, we identified the relationship between a force vector acting on a lever arm at an angle and the moment arm that it creates. Based on the force angle, we noticed how different angles lead to differing moment arm lengths between the line of force and the axis of rotation.

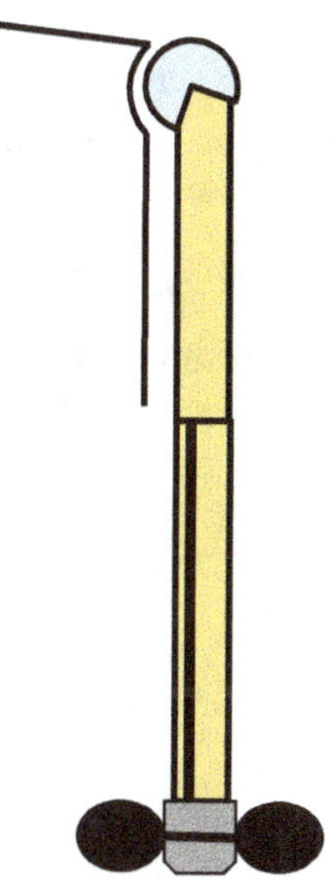

Whenever a force is applied at a 90-degree angle to a lever, that force can produce rotation of that lever around an axis of rotation. However, in situations where the force vector is not at a 90-degree force angle to the lever, it won't solely provide rotary Motion but will also assist in other functions, which we shall now explore.

Illustration showcasing the Shoulder joint Complex alongside a 10-pound dumbbell being held onto as an "external" load.

Note: This example will only consider the relationship between the external load (10-pound dumbbell) in hand to the Deltoids line of pull.

Scenario 1: Determining basic forces acting on the Shoulder Joint Complex based on what's been covered until now.

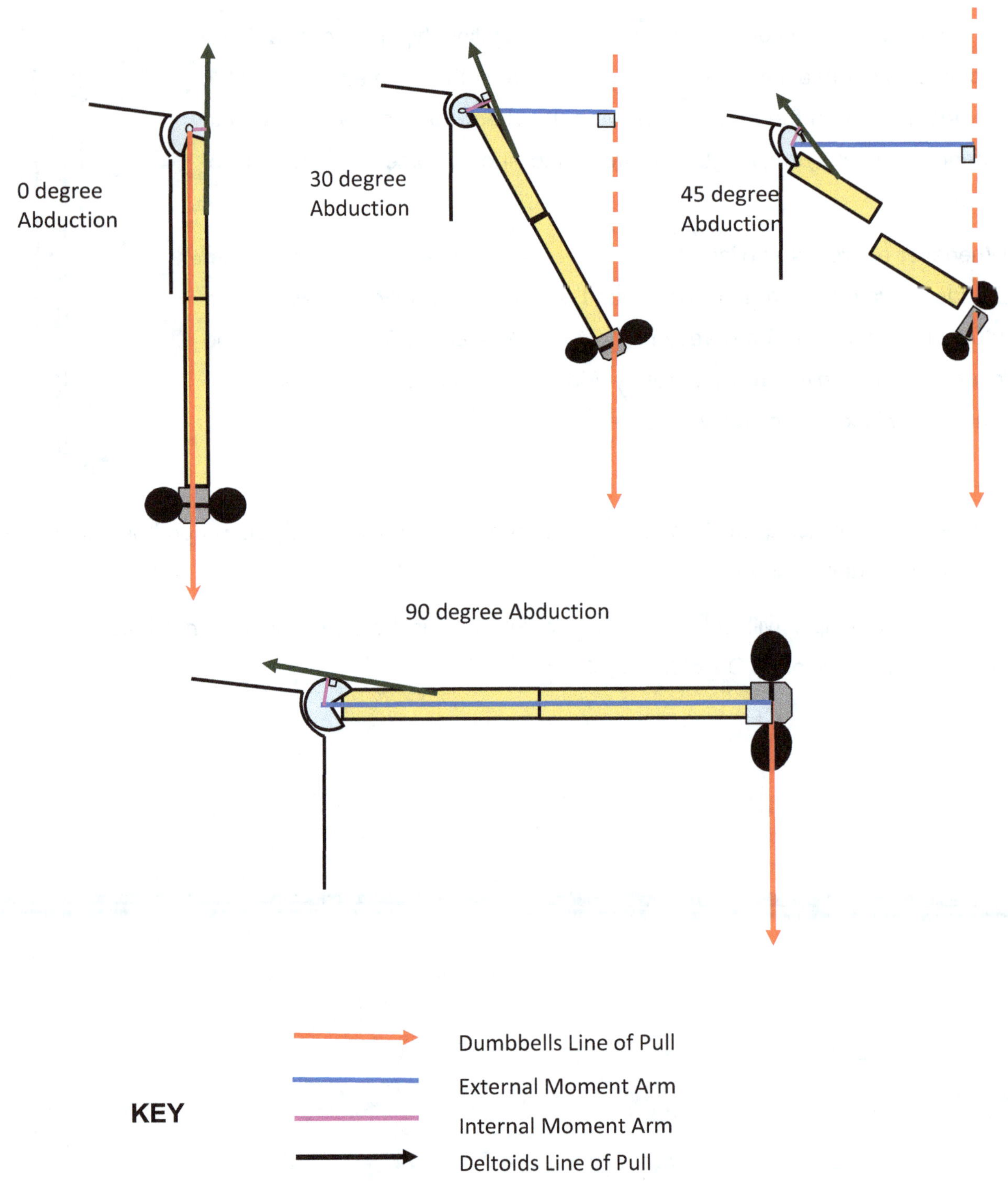

The above four scenarios showcase the relationship between external forces and internal forces acting on the shoulder joint at four different joint angles, 0 degrees, 30 degrees, 45 degrees, and 90 degrees of shoulder abduction.

Let's start exploring each joint angle, the ability of the external load to produce external torque, and the ability of the internal deltoid force to produce internal torque.

To begin with, at 0 degrees of shoulder abduction, the 10-pound dumbbell remains 10 pounds. Its mass accelerates at 9.8m/s^2 downwards. Thus, the force the dumbbell exerts would be F = M.A = 10lb x 9.8m/s^2 = 98N

98N is the external force.

At 0 degrees of abduction, 98N remains 98N as the external force, but the amount of torque that this external force is creating at the shoulder joint is negligible. Look at the distance between the line of force (dashed line going towards the shoulder joints axis) and the shoulder joints axis.

There is no moment arm for the 98N force to create any torque around the shoulder joint. In this scenario, the dumbbell is just chilling.

However, when checking out the deltoids line of pull. We see that the Deltoid has a moment arm (a small one) between its line of pull and the shoulder joint's axis of rotation. If needed, the Deltoid can exert small force to simply ABduct the shoulder. Let's say that the internal moment is 0.01 m. Hence the Deltoid can produce the least force possible to ABduct the shoulder.

At 45 degrees of ABduction, 98N external force created by the dumbbell remains 98N, but the amount of torque it can produce at the shoulder joint now increases. This external force can create shoulder ADDuction torque at the shoulder joint due to a longer moment arm present.

Let's say the moment arm is 0.30m (30cm) away from the line of the external force. This increases the torque experienced to 98N x 0.30 m = 29.4 Nm of shoulder ADDuction torque.

Coming to the internal force produced by the Deltoid, we can see that the internal moment arm of the Deltoid's line of pull has increased relative to its internal amount arm at 0 degrees of ABduction.

Let's say the moment arm length is now 0.02 m. This would require the Deltoid to produce an internal force of 1470N to maintain the shoulder joint at 45 degrees of ABduction. However, to have the shoulder ABduct continuously, it would have to produce forces greater than 1470N.

As the shoulder joint moves into 90 degrees of shoulder abduction, we immediately must understand that the deltoids have been able to produce sufficient forces to create enough internal torque to overcome the external torque created at the shoulder joint by the dumbbell (98N of force).

At 90 degrees of shoulder ABduction, we now have the external force acting on the arm at 90 degrees. This would produce a 90-degree force angle!

We know that whenever there is a 90-degree force angle, the length of the moment arm is the longest. 98N can now create the greatest amount of torque relative to other joint angles covered.

For instance, if the length of the moment arm is now 0.50 m, the external torque created will now become 98N x 0.50 m = 49Nm

Let's check out what's happening internally. We see that the deltoid moment arm to create internal torque had reduced in length relative to when the shoulder joint was abducted to 45 degrees.

A reduction in moment arm length indicates that the deltoids had entered a disadvantage significantly when the external moment arm increased.

For instance, if the internal moment arm is now 0.016m, the internal force required to hold static at 90 degrees of ABduction = 3062.5N (49 Nm / 0.016 m).

At this point in the joint's ABduction ROM, the person holding the dumbbell will experience the most resistance. This is one of the reasons why the Dumbbell Lateral Raise Exercise feels hardest at the topmost point in the range of Motion.

LET'S NOW DIVE INTO COMPONENT FORCES.

As seen in force angles, a force will have the greatest rotary effect when the angle between the line of force and the lever arm is 90 degrees. This is because a 90-degree force angle can cause the highest amount of torque around an axis relative to any other force angle.

A force angle to a segment other than 90 degrees would participate in rotation and other functions. We shall have two significant components whenever a force acts upon a segment at an angle other than 90 degrees: the rotary and translatory components. The rotary component will always be considered perpendicular to the lever arm, whereas the translatory component will always be regarded as parallel to the lever arm.

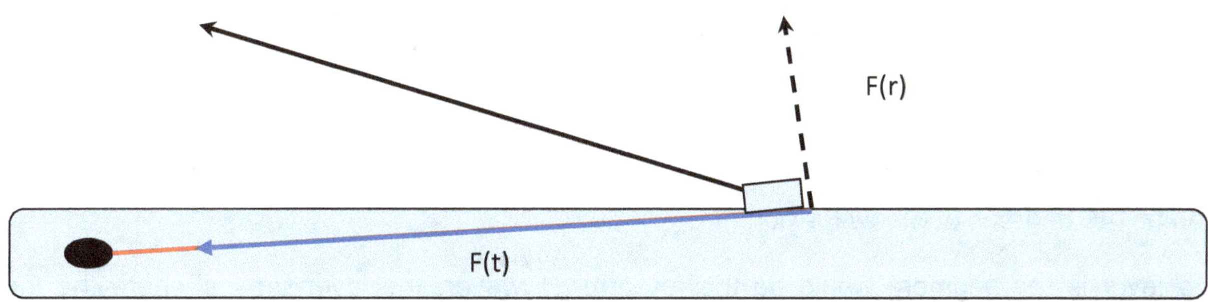

The following illustration projects a static segment with a force vector running at an angle away from the segment.

Given that the force angle is not 90 degrees, it cannot produce pure rotation of the segment around the axis of the rotation.

Thus we can divide this force vector into two of its components. F(r) and F(t) are the rotary and translatory forces, respectively.

F(r), the rotary force works on the lever arm to produce pure rotation because it creates a 90-degree force angle with the lever arm of the segment.

F(t), the translatory force works on the lever arm to produce translatory Motion as it overlaps the lever arm. It lies parallel to the lever arm, which works to push the segment into the axis of rotation.

In this illustration, most of the force created by the original force vector creates translatory Motion relative to some rotary motion. This is because the force vector f(t) is longer relative to f(r).

FORCE COMPONENTS IN THE HUMAN BODY

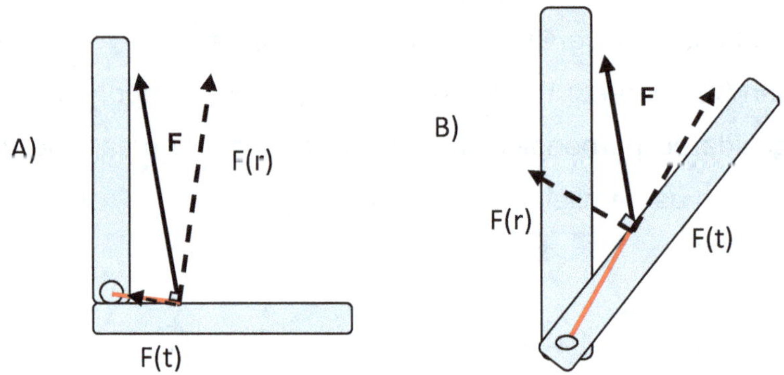

In the above two examples, the elbow joint is first seen at 90 degrees of Elbow Flexion (A) and then at 145 degrees of Elbow Flexion (B).

The lever is the segment would be the forearm. However, the lever arm is where the force vector acts; the line between the joint's axis of rotation and the point of application of the force vector (F) is the lever arm.

Illustration A: We see that the (F) acts upon the lever arm diagonally, creating two components of force, F(r) and F(t). F(r) would be considered the rotary component because it is placed at 90 degrees to the lever arm. Thus this force vector would solely assist in rotation around the joint's axis. Moreover, F(t) would be considered the translatory component because it is placed exactly in line with the lever arm. This force vector assists in compression, i.e., pressing two bony segments together. In this case, the compressive force is considered stabilizing, as it keeps the joint together.

However, in the current scenario, we see that the rotary component F(r) is longer relative to the translatory component. This increases rotary torque at the elbow joint, causing elbow flexion.

Illustration B: We see that the elbow has greater elbow flexion. The relationships between the force components thus have changed. The force vector F is applied to the lever arm because it is at an angle other than 90 degrees, leading to it having two components. The rotary component F(r) and the translatory component F(t). In this scenario, we have a longer translatory component relative to the rotary component. Here, the translatory component does not achieve compression but is a distraction force. A distraction force is a force that leads to a separation between two bony segments. The relative proportions between the two force components result in rotation alongside distraction.

FORCE COMPONENTS *OF EXTERNAL FORCES*

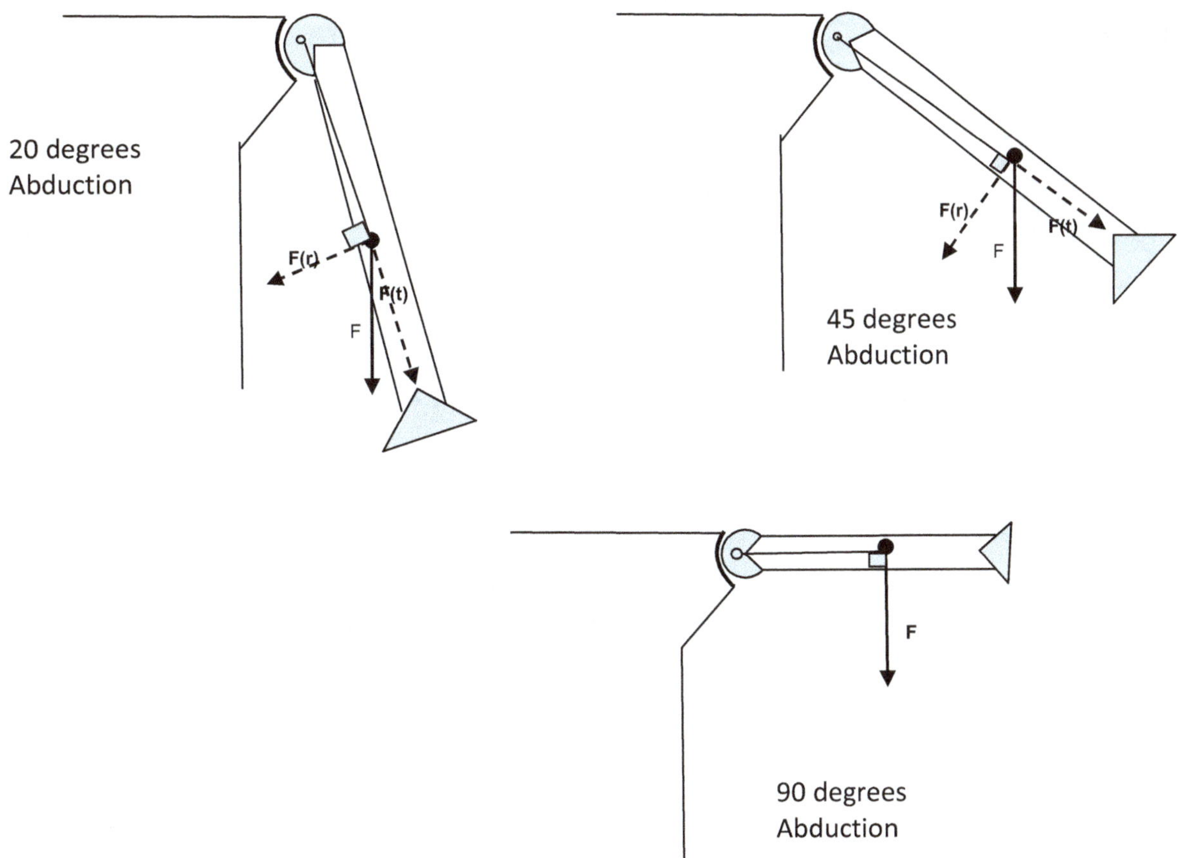

The above illustrations show the shoulder joint at three angles of ABduction, 20, 45, and 90 degrees. The lever is the humerus, and the lever arm is the distance between the shoulder axis of rotation and the point of the force application. The force acting on the humerus is directed downwards towards Gravity. The point of application would be around the center of mass of the humerus. The Force Vector (F) is always going to be downward when considering Gravity.

At 20 degrees of shoulder abduction, the force vector F is divided into its components, F(r) and F(t). F(r) is the rotation component, and F(t) is the translatory component. The rotational component is shorter relative to the translatory component at this degree of shoulder abduction.

The translatory component becomes a distraction component that works to separate the congruency between the two articulating surfaces of the joint.

Given that there is no constraint, the humerus will tend to rotate and go towards the direction of Gravity.

At 90 degrees of shoulder abduction, the magnitude of the force exerted at the point of application will solely produce rotation around the shoulder joint, taking the humerus into adduction. There would be no translation component due to no force vector passing through the joint axis.

INTRODUCTION TO LEVER SYSTEMS

As previously mentioned, a lever can be any segment that is made to rotate around an axis. This axis can also be called a fulcrum.

A lever system is established when two opposing forces are applied simultaneously to the lever to create opposing torques (an effect of the force used).

Think of the forearm as a lever, a bony segment in the human body. The biceps produce internal forces that create internal torque to oppose external forces applied by a dumbbell, producing external torque at the elbow joint.

This creates a lever system.

Thus, to have a lever system, we need two important elements:

- Two opposing forces
- An axis of rotation.

Opposing Forces: To create opposing torques around an axis of rotation, there need to be forces acting on a segment at differing lengths from the axis of rotation.

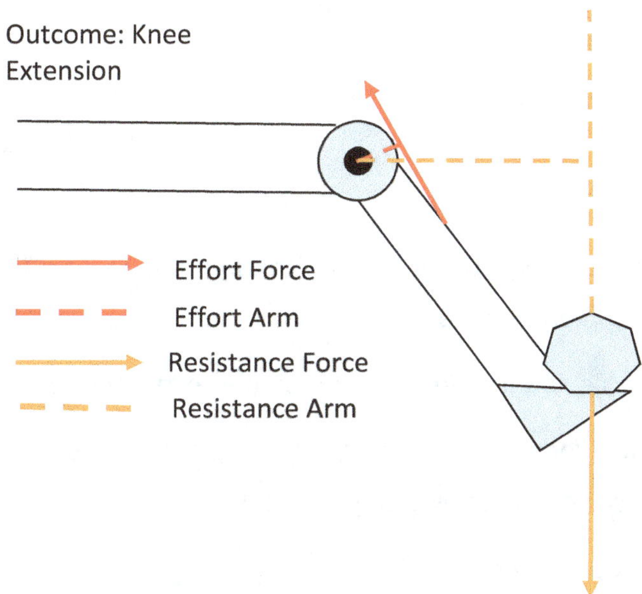

The above illustration showcases the relationship between two opposing forces and the end outcome, which results in knee extension.

During knee extension, the quadriceps produce sufficient internal force to oppose and win over the external force applied at the ankle joint in the way of a dumbbell.

Internal force is being produced to create torque at the knee joint to offset and win over the torque created by the external force placed on the dumbbell.

The force that creates the winning torque can be called the Effort Force.

In comparison, the force that resists the effort force but doesn't succeed is called the resistance force.

Things change once the situation is reversed.

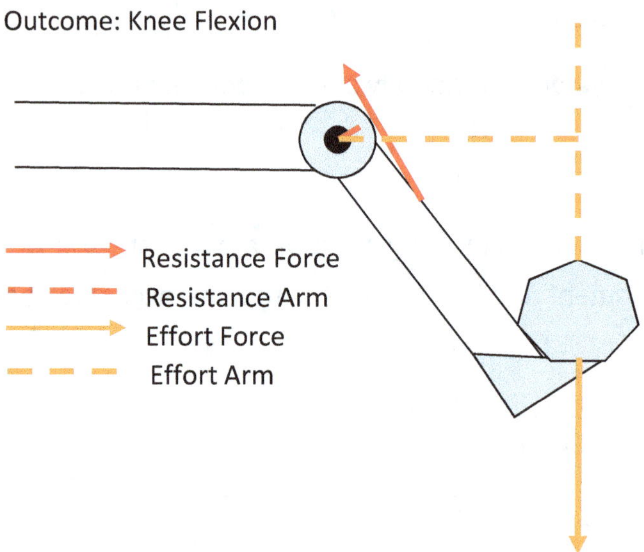

Suppose, instead of there being 10 lbs on the ankle, there is now 30 lbs, or the quadriceps cannot produce sufficient internal force.

The result leads to "knee flexion torque" created by the external force.

In this scenario, the effort force is the external force placed on the ankle, and the resistance force is the eccentric force produced by the quadriceps.

An easier way to remember this concept:

The effort force always wins the battle.

The resistance force does not win the battle.

EFFORT AND RESISTANCE ARMS

The respective moment arms from the knee joint to the line of force denote "effort" and "resistance" arms.

 Notice how the effort and resistance arm switch, as a result, changes from knee extension to flexion.

Types of Lever Systems

1. A First Class Lever System

A system where the effort and resistance arms are on two opposite sides of the pivot point. For example, A seesaw.

Having the effort and resistance forces equidistant from the pivot point is optional. This is very rare in the human body. Resistance force and effort force are equidistant from the pivot point.

A longer resistance arm relative to a shorter effort arm due to a change in the pivot point's position.

A shorter resistance arm relative to a longer effort arm due to a change in the pivot point's position.

A common example of a 1st class lever system is the relationship between the Triceps acting on the humerus and the external force acting on the forearm.

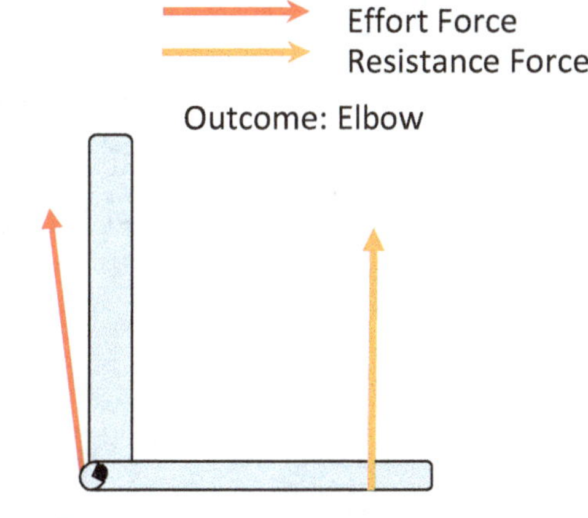

In this illustration, the Triceps act upon Ulna to create elbow extension torque to oppose elbow flexion torque produced by an external force (cable). This makes up a first-class lever system due to the orientation of the forces relative to the pivot point.

In the scenario where the elbow goes into flexion due to a greater external force, the resistance force would now be the Triceps line of pull, and the effort force becomes the cable pulling the forearm into elbow flexion.

2. A *Second Class* Lever System

In a 2nd class lever, the effort and the resistance force always act on the other side of a pivot point. The proportions of the effort arm, the resistance arm, and the net torque created by the forces acting on the segment will decide whether the lever system is considered a 2nd class system or a 3rd class system.

In a 2nd class system, the resistance force always lies in between the effort and the pivot point.

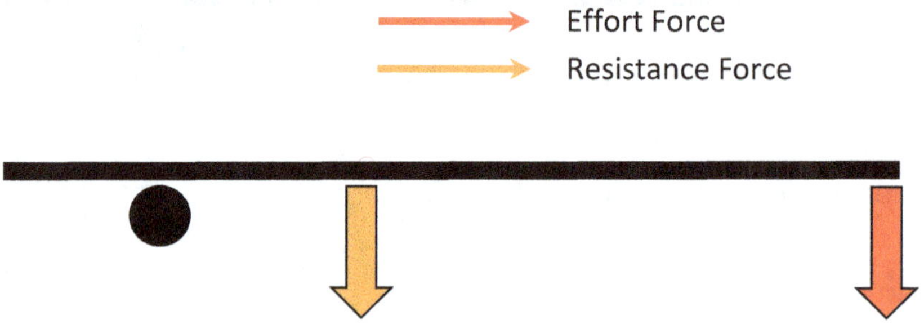

To figure out the lever system, we must first calculate the net torque created around the pivot point.

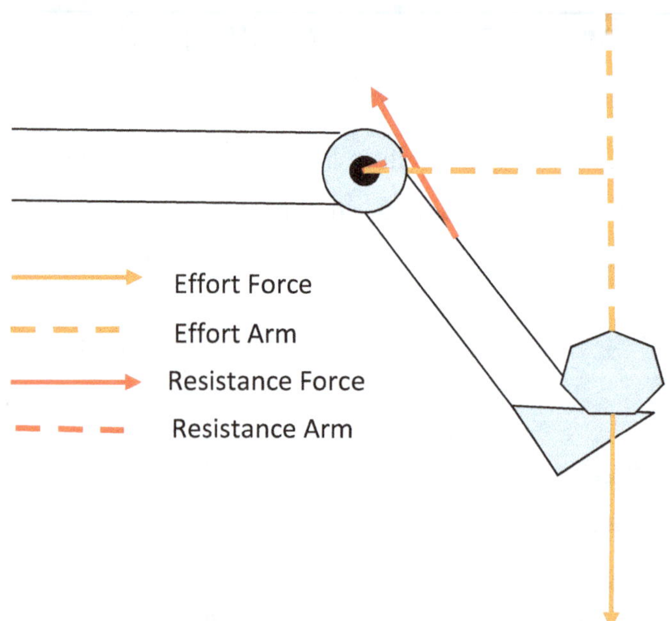

Here let's make a few assumptions to clearly understand the concept that differentiate a 2nd class lever from 3rd class lever.

In the given example, assume that the lower limb alongside the 10-pound dumbbell on the ankle produces an external force of 250N. The moment arm between the knee joints axis and the resultant line of force is assumed to be 0.10 m

The torque created by the external force = + 250 N X 0.10 m = + 25 Nm of Knee flexion torque.

Assume that the quadriceps are producing - 1000 N of internal force at 0.02 m from the knee's axis of rotation.

This suggests the internal torque creating knee extension by the quadriceps = - 1000N X 0.02 m = - 20 Nm.

The resulting torque

 = 25Nm - 20Nm

= 5 Nm in the direction of Knee Flexion.

In this case, the quadricep cannot produce sufficient internal forces to oppose knee flexion torque created by an external force.

 In this scenario, the winner is the external force; thus, the effort force is the force exerted on the limb by the dumbbell and the weight of the limb as a whole. The quadriceps line of pull becomes the resistance force.

The Quadriceps are still working. It means that the quadriceps are still functioning to resist knee flexion by contracting eccentrically.

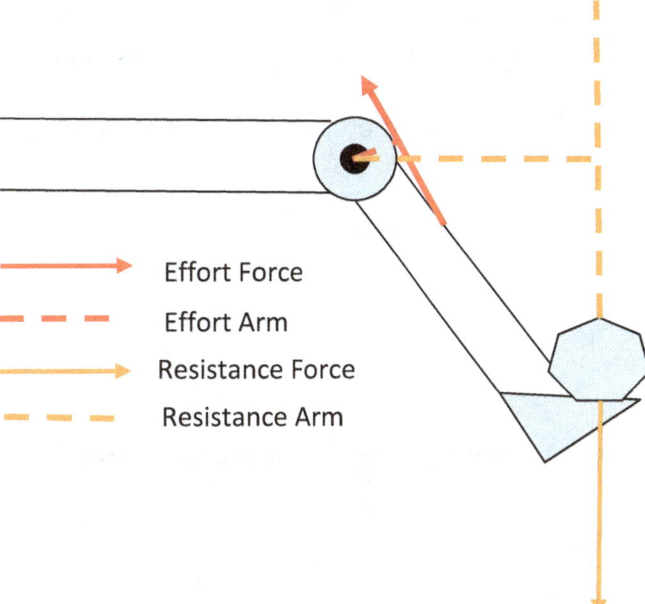

3. A *Third Class* **Lever**

Continuing the example presented above, suppose the quadriceps can produce a lot more force to oppose external forces created by knee flexion torque.

Let's assume that the Quadriceps are now producing - 1500N of internal force, 0.02 m from the axis.

Knee extension torque produced: - 30Nm of torque

Resulting torque at the knee joint: -30Nm + 25Nm   = -5 Nm

The quadriceps could overcome knee flexion torque by producing sufficient internal forces to create above and beyond the required torque. The net outcome would be knee extension against external forces: Gravity and the dumbbell on the ankle.

In this scenario, the effort force is the quadriceps line of pull between the joint's axis, the resistance force exerted by Gravity, and the dumbbell acting on the ankle.

Mechanical Advantage

What is a mechanical advantage, and why should we be bothered about having an advantage?

Google defines advantage as "Something that puts you in a better position than other people.

Although we are not considering people in this text, we need to realize that Mechanical Advantage is the ability of a lever system to either be efficient or inefficient. It is based on the ratio of effort and resistance arms.

Mechanical Advantage = Effort Arm/Resistance Arm

We explored that an effort arm is the shortest perpendicular distance between a lever's axis and the effort forces acting on the lever. Moreover, a resistance arm is the shortest perpendicular distance between a lever's axis and the resistance forces acting on the lever.

A mechanical ratio greater than one denotes that the effort arm is longer than the resistance arm.

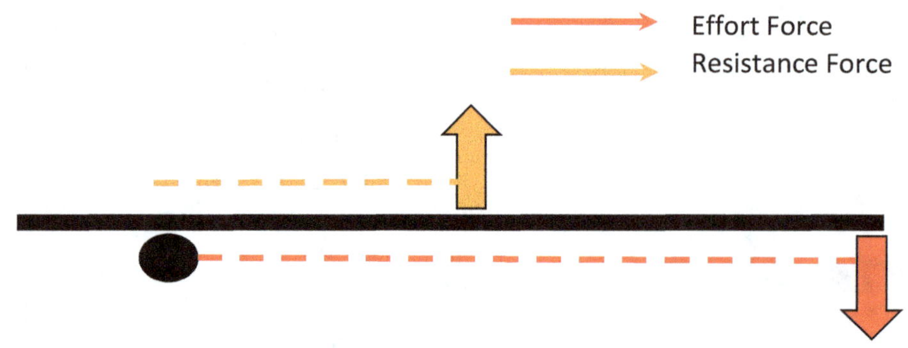

In this example, the lever is mechanically efficient.

Effort arm = 20 inches

Resistance arm = 12 inches

Efficiency: 1.667, which provides an advantage.

The advantage is that the magnitude of effort force required to create torque around the axis would be lesser than the magnitude of resistance force required to create torque around the axis. This is achieved due to a longer moment arm for the effort force relative to the moment arm of the resistance force.

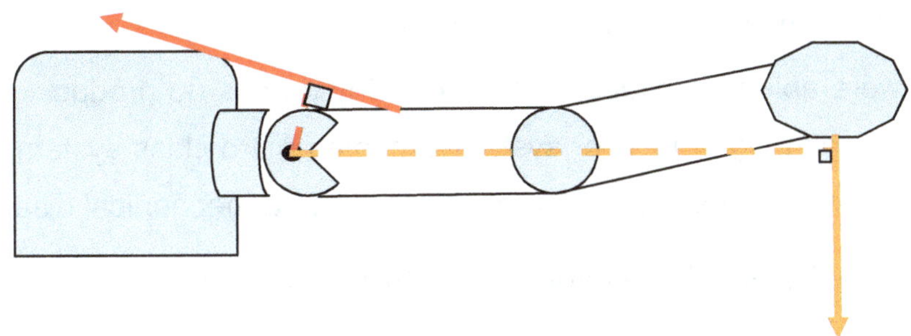

The above example showcases an individual performing dumbbell flies in an attempt to train the Pectoralis Major Muscle.

We see the 10 lb dumbbell acting downward on the forearm and the Pecs line of pull on the humerus.

The resistance arm here is the internal moment arm of the pecs, whereas the effort arm here is the external moment arm between the axis and the line of external force.

This makes a 2nd class lever system due to the placement of the resistance force between the joint's axis of rotation and the effort force.

The 10-pound dumbbell provides 98N of force downwards in the line of Gravity. The pecs have to overcome shoulder ABduction torque by producing sufficient internal forces.

Say the length of the external moment arm is 0.30 m, and the length of the internal moment arm is 0.05 m.

The amount of torque the Pecs have to overcome here is 29Nm. Thus, it must create at least 588N of force (29.4Nm/0.05m).

Due to the resistance arm being only 0.05m relative to the effort arm of 0.30m, the external force is at a mechanical advantage to produce ABduction torque at the shoulder.

It requires only 98N of force, whereas the pecs require to produce 588N of force to maintain this position and would require much more than 588N of force to overcome the influence of external force.

The amount of mechanical advantage the external load receives depends on a lot of factors as well.

- The length of the external moment arm
- The force angle of the external force
- The length of the internal moment arm
- The line of pull of the internal force-producing unit

In case, the Pecs were able to produce more force. Say it ends up producing 700N of internal force. In this scenario, although the lever system becomes a 3rd class system (due to the effort force now being the pec's internal force), the pecs are still at a mechanical disadvantage.

The pecs must produce 700N of force to offset just 98N of external force.

Mechanical Advantage Ratio: 0.05m/0.30m = 0.16

In the human body, most muscles work via a shorter moment arm relative to a longer external moment arm. To produce force by contracting concentrically, the muscle works with a shorter moment arm. It thus would require to produce of higher forces to offset a weaker external force placed further from a joint's axis of rotation. This reality creates a mechanical disadvantage in a variety of skeletal muscle groups.

An advantage to a mechanically disadvantaged/inefficient lever system?

We saw how the biceps acts in a third-class lever system at a mechanical disadvantage relative to an advantage for the external load placed further away from the joint's axis of rotation. Thus, the muscle's required force to create the winning torque must be larger than the force placed externally on the limb.

However, the following illustration showcases a peculiar characteristic of such lever systems.

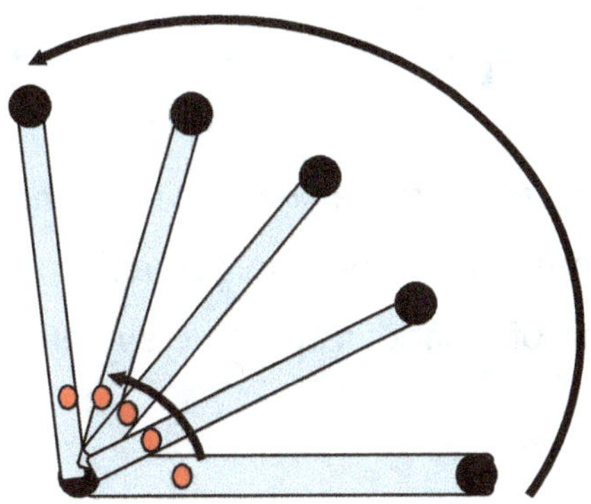

Look what happens to the distance traveled by the dots as the bicep flexes the elbow joint. The distance traveled by the external black dots (an external segment) is far more than that of the internal red dots (point of Bicep Attachment).

This means that a smaller range of Motion traveled by the red dot produces a large range externally in terms of degree.

This is an advantage for the Biceps.

Moreover, the distance covered by the point where the muscle attaches and the external segment occurs simultaneously. This means the external segment is moving at a much faster speed.

For instance, in 1 second, the external segment covers 10 inches for every 2 inches covered by the point where the Biceps attaches.

MISCELLANEOUS **TOPICS**

1. CONCURRENT FORCE SYSTEMS

A resultant force vector is formed by force lines intersecting a common point of application but may have diverging action lines. When such forces act upon this common point of application, the forces are said to be a part of a concurrent force system.

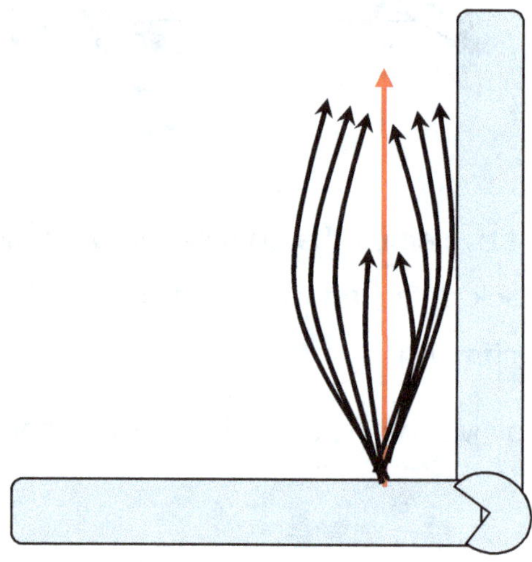

This illustration showcases the line of pull of the Hamstrings as it works to extend the knee. The Hamstrings are composed of three main heads that cross the hip and knee joints and one that only crosses the knee joint. In response to the external force causing knee extension torque, the hamstrings work to flex the knee.

The resultant line of pull of the hamstrings is seen in red. Although we see just one prominent line of pull, each muscle fiber has its force vector, creating a resultant pull line causing knee flexion. This makes a concurrent force system as multiple vectors work on one application point.

As the hamstrings contract, it works to generate forces on both the segments it attaches to. However, the lighter segment (Tibia and Fibula) are the ones that can move towards the heavier and more stable segment (The Pelvis).

2. DIVERGENT *LINES OF ACTION*

This illustration showcases the line of action of each quadricep head acting working to create knee extension torque. We see the Vastus Medialis, Vastus Lateralis, and Superior Rectus Femoris. The resultant force of the Vastus Medialis and the Vastus Lateralis Muscle are shown. When these two head contract together, we have a resultant vector that runs between them, creating pure knee extension. Mf is a quadriceps line of pull in this example.

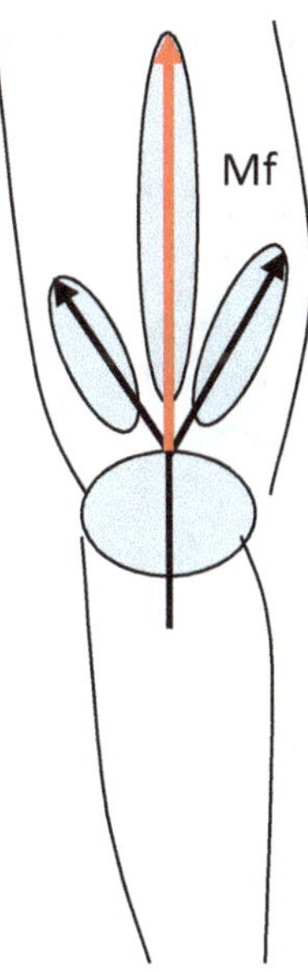

3. ANATOMICAL *PULLEYS*

Pulleys are tools used to change the direction in which a force is applied. It plays an important role in redirecting forces.

This illustration demonstrates a pulley system outside of the human body. The wheel remains fixed while being attached to a segment. A cord tends to span around the wheel to redirect the force.

This pulley system has only one wheel around which a force is redirected. In this scenario, the magnitude of force remains the same on both sides of the wheel.

In the human body, instead of having wheels that redirect forces, we have bony landmarks, ligaments, cartilage, and skeletal muscle that allow the redirection of forces.

In most instances, the cords are the tendons that attach muscles to bones as they cross a joint. A tendon may wrap around a pulley wheel, creating a pulley system that assists in redirecting forces.

Pulleys in the human body can be considered "Anatomic Pulleys." Not only do such pulleys alter the direction of force, but they also assist in increasing the amount of torque the muscle can create if there were no such pulleys in the body. Due to the change in force direction produced by the muscle wrapping over the "bony landmark," there is an increase in the internal moment arm distance between the joint's axis of rotation and the muscle's line of pull.

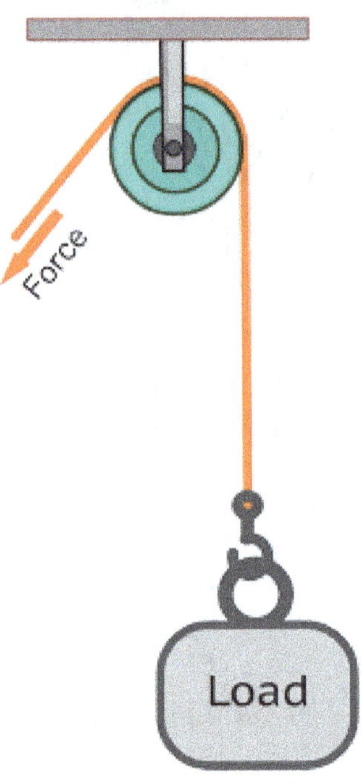

Example of an anatomical pulley in the body: The Patella forming the Patello-Femoral Joint.

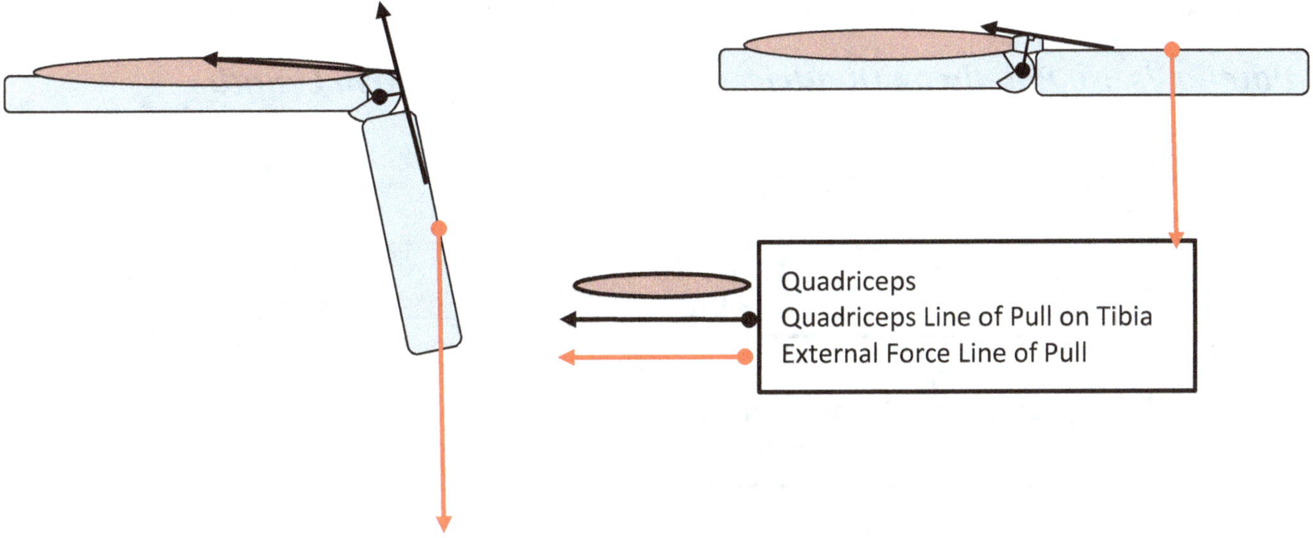

In the above illustration, we see the Patella acting as an anatomical pulley, which allows the force to be redirected by the quadriceps on the lower leg (Tibia).

Not only does the Patella play an important role as an anatomical pulley, but it also works as an anatomical CAM. A CAM plays the role of providing a mechanical advantage to a force-producing object.

Although we have not explored muscle physiology yet, let's assume that skeletal muscles have the potential to produce greater mechanical tension (force production) in their mid-range relative to longer or shorter lengths. In the illustration to the left, we have the quadriceps in their long to mid-range. In this position, the quadriceps can produce the required tension to oppose knee flexion torque caused by external forces. Although the internal moment arm is short in this scenario, the quadriceps can get away with reduced tension production because it is in a stronger length. Moreover, the shorter external moment arm reduces the amount of knee flexion torque the quadriceps must overcome.

But look what happens when the knee is completely extended at 0 degrees knee flexion. The external moment arm increases relative to the previous illustration. Moreover, the quadriceps is now at a shorter length as well. These two factors reduce the ability of the quadriceps to produce sufficient tension to oppose knee flexion torque created by the external load. However, due to the CAM-like effects of the Patella, we have increased the internal moment arm length of the quadriceps. This occurs because the quadricep tension wraps around the Patella, which also redirects forces produced by the quadriceps. The quadriceps may not have the best advantage to build higher tension but now work through a longer moment arm. We know the influence of a moment arm on the amount of torque that can be produced.

Patella Vs. No Patella on Quadricep Internal Moment Arm Length

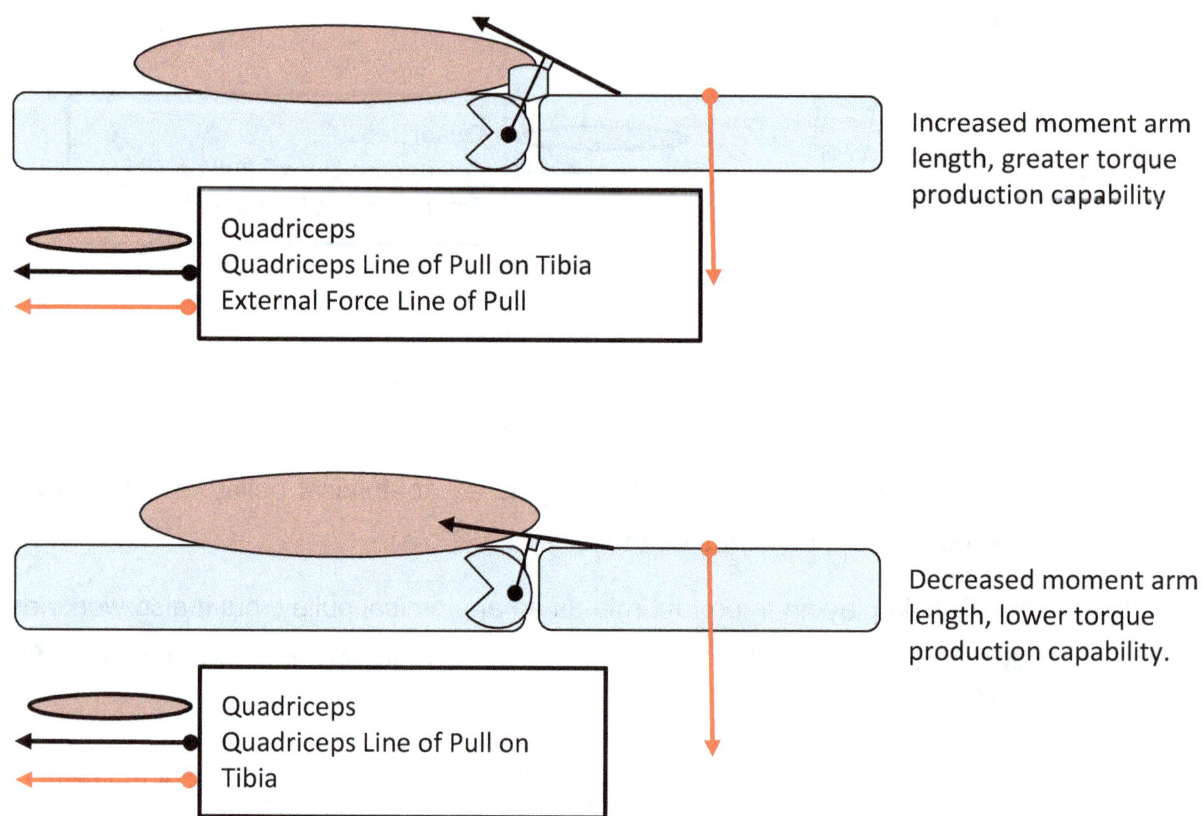

4. *MUSCLE LINE OF PULL* AND *HYPERTROPHY: IS THERE A RELATIONSHIP?*

Muscle hypertrophy refers to the increase in the size of individual muscle fibers. As mentioned earlier, each fiber contains smaller units called Sarcomeres. Muscle fibers get larger due to adding sarcomeres in parallel (one on top of the other) or series (Like a continuous chain of sarcomeres). As a muscle hypertrophies, it receives a mechanical advantage in terms of an optimal line of pull on the lever arm.

Let's take the example of the Biceps.

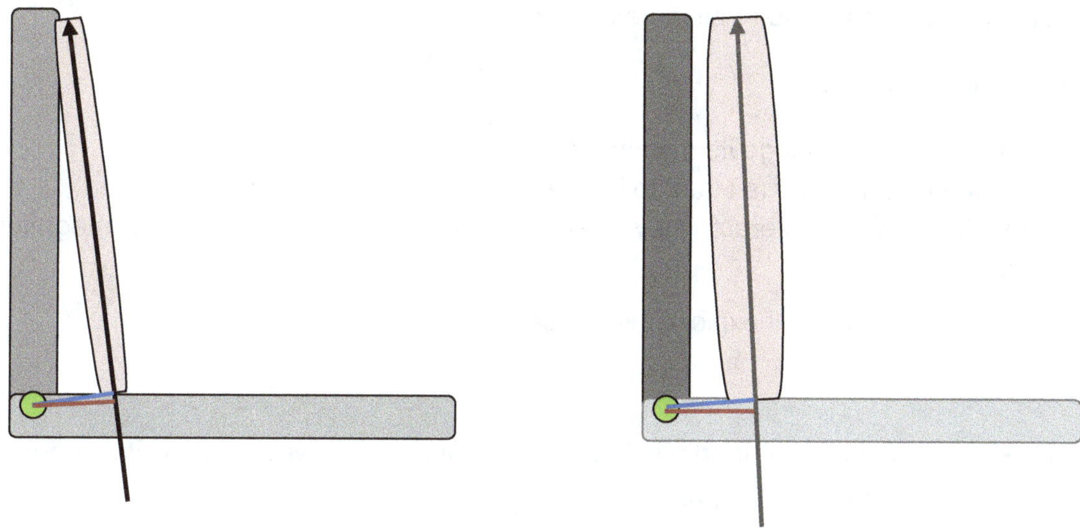

The current illustration shows that the biceps have grown in size in response to a training stimulus. The force angle between the lever (the forearm) and the point of force application increase from being less perpendicular to slightly closer to being perpendicular. This improves the biceps line of pull on the lower arm. We know now that as the force angle approaches closer to 90 degrees, the length of a moment arm increases. Since we are talking about internal forces in this example, a longer internal moment arm can increase the amount of torque generated. This is one reason a bigger muscle is stronger than a smaller one.

5. *FORCES* WE EXPERIENCE

Let's consider re-visiting what force is to distinguish between different forces acting upon us.

Force is a push or a pull. This means when a force acts on an object, it results in a simple push of one thing on another or a pull of one thing on another. Force is an entity that either produces motion, halts motion, or changes the direction of motion (Paraphrased from "Biomechanics of Human Movement" by Barney).

Throughout this book, we covered external forces and internal forces that tend to act on the body. We mainly focused on the external force, Gravity, and the internal force, Muscular Tension. However, this section will briefly touch upon other contact forces that are usually not visible but add to the resistance training experience.

What did Newton's Law Say?

1) An object will not change its motion unless a force acts on it.
2) The force on an object is equal to its mass times its acceleration.
3) When two objects interact, they apply forces to each other of equal magnitude and opposite direction.

Based on the 1st law, we shall explore the concept of:

5.1 Inertia

Inertia is resistance to change. Inertia is the property of mass, or you can call it a property of an object. The property of an object that resists change is termed inertia.

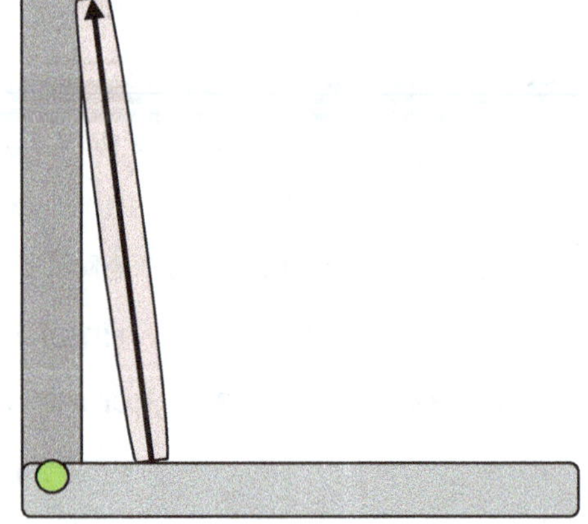

For instance, assume that the forearm is perpendicular to the floor in this illustration. To maintain elbow flexion, our biceps have to produce the required torque to oppose the external torque imposed by gravity acting on the forearm.

This position can be sustained if the biceps can produce sufficient force. To disrupt the equilibrium, there has to be some change. Either the biceps may have to overcome the torque created by the external force, or the external force may have to increase in magnitude or be applied at a distance further from the joint's axis to overcome the torque created by the biceps.

Just as an object at rest tends to be at rest, an object in motion tends to be in motion. Hence the moment the biceps can create more torque by increasing mechanical tension production or the magnitude of external force increases/is placed further from the joints axis, the elbow will want to flex or extend respectively. To stop this added motion, there needs to be something that prevents it from continuous movement. This "something" could be bony structures, skeletal muscle, or connective tissues that span the joint.

Inertia is resistance to change, forces are required to break the equilibrium when the forearm is parallel to the floor, and forces are also required to resist the urge of the forearm to keep being in motion.

Something to also consider is, Inertia is NOT a force but the effects of a force acting on an object.

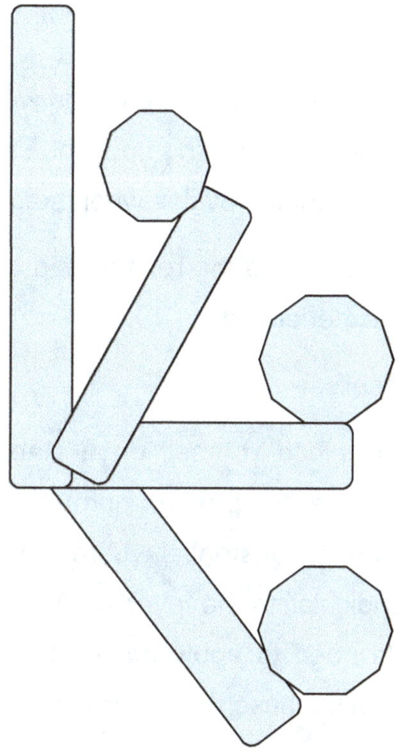

This illustration showcases a traditionally performed Bicep Curl exercise, where the external force on the lower arm creates elbow extension torque at the shoulder. Thus to overcome this torque, the Elbow Flexors have to produce sufficient forces that create flexion torque at the shoulder.

However, let's explore what happens when the dumbbell is made to accelerate upward quicker than usual. Due to this change in speed, the "load" on the arm is not the same relative to having a more controlled tempo. The dumbbell still has mass and is still directed toward gravity. Still, the upward acceleration causes the dumbbell to counter the gravitational pull on the dumbbell, which reduces the load placed on the arm.

We see individuals use momentum, increasing the arm's tempo in space. This reduces the load placed on the arm and hence elbow extension torque at that point. Thus, this reduces the amount of torque the biceps may need to produce to overcome elbow extension torque.

As tempo increases, the inertial effects increase as well. The urge to lift the dumbbell as fast as possible will make it want to keep traveling upwards unless brakes are applied, i.e., to resist it— the amount of torque the dumbbell provides when stagnant may vary.

The following continuum showcases the relationship between the inertial effects of free weights and the amount of torque experienced.

You could try this for yourself.

Take a 5kg dumbbell and place yourself on a stable surface to perform Bicep Curls. Start repping the weight with a faster tempo than normal. You would soon realize that the load feels different. You may feel nothing substantial where the resistance probably is the greatest (when the line of force is perpendicular to the lever arm). You may feel greater resistance at the end ranges, where you would need to apply brakes to your arm, which is susceptible to inertial effects. Brakes are required because the lower arm would want to keep going in the direction of force application, as it has not only its own mass but also the added mass of the dumbbell, which is susceptible to inertial effects.

Take the same 5kg dumbbell and control the tempo at which you perform each rep. You would notice how the resistance your muscles need to overcome reduces at the end ranges but increases at the mid-range. This is one of the resistance profiles that free weight provides us with as long as the rep tempo is well under control.

The above pointers cover the basic concepts relating to inertia and its effects.

5.2 Friction

Frictional forces come into play when two or more objects/segments come in contact. Think of friction as a force that prevents objects in contact from slipping away from each another.

The concept of friction arises from Newton's Third Law of Motion which states when two objects interact, they apply forces to each other of equal magnitude and opposite direction. Contact between two objects refers to them being in contact with one another. The force vector's direction depends on the direction in which the objects in contact move. Friction always tends to oppose the motion of the objects. In the illustration below, the two blocks in contact with one another want to slide apart in opposite directions. However, the force opposing that from happening is Friction, which works to create forces in the opposite direction in which each block moves.

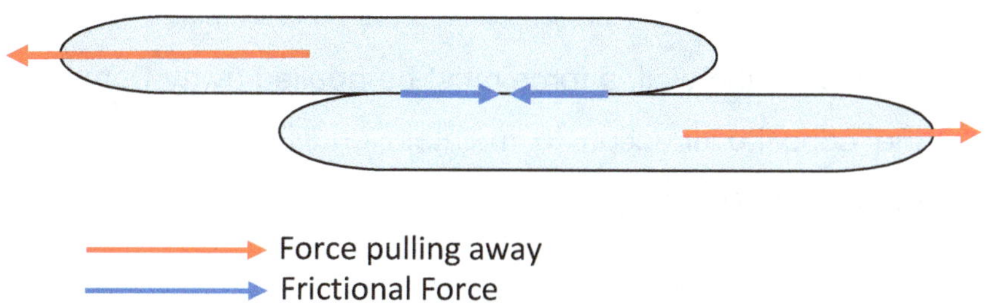

Friction allows us to walk, run and get to places using modes of transportation.

Moreover, friction also exists within our joints. Bony structures, connective tissues, and muscles may come into contact with one another during movement, which creates friction to tend to oppose such movements. For instance, there could be friction between a tendon and a bone over which the tendon passes.

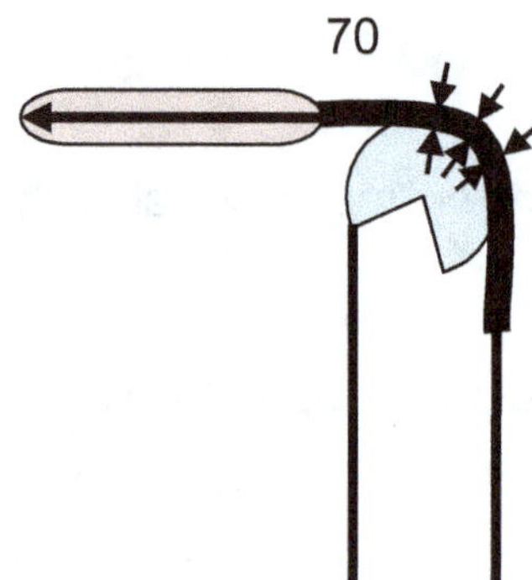

In the following illustration, we see a tendon on a muscle attaching to a limb as it rolls over a bony segment. As the muscle pulls on its attachment, the tendon may pass over the bony segment creating contact between the two. This leads to the development of friction between the two contact surfaces.

Frictional forces are at play during a wall sit:

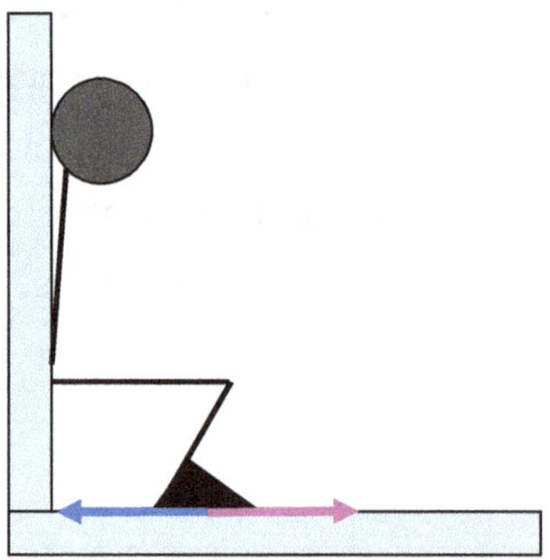

For the individual to stay stuck to the wall, a force must be applied away from the ground, which creates opposition in the opposite direction to maintain equilibrium. The force opposing the forward force on the ground is Friction.

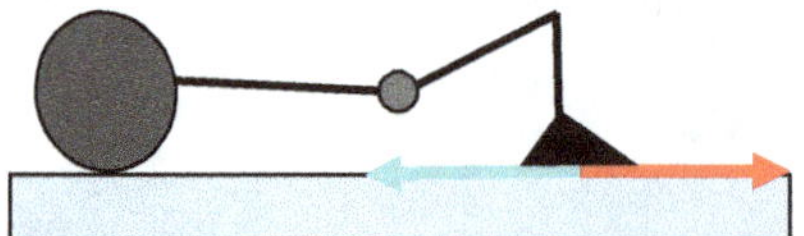

The concept applies during a Hip Thrust. As force is exerted onto the floor, there would also be forces exerted linearly parallel to the ground, creating a reaction force in the opposite direction called Friction.

How frictional forces may provide different experiences during two popular chest exercises.

The Bench Press Vs. The Dumbbell Press: What movement pattern requires the Triceps to produce force?

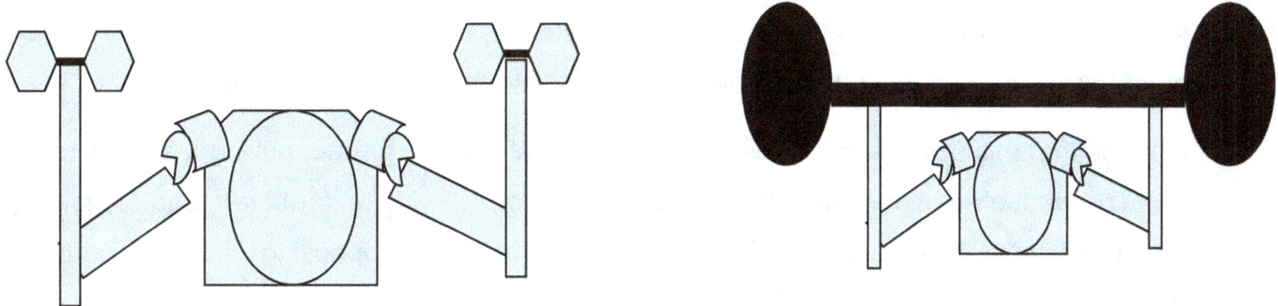

In this illustration, we will analyze two forces acting externally on the body: Gravitational Force and Frictional Force.

Let's first analyze the Dumbbell Press:

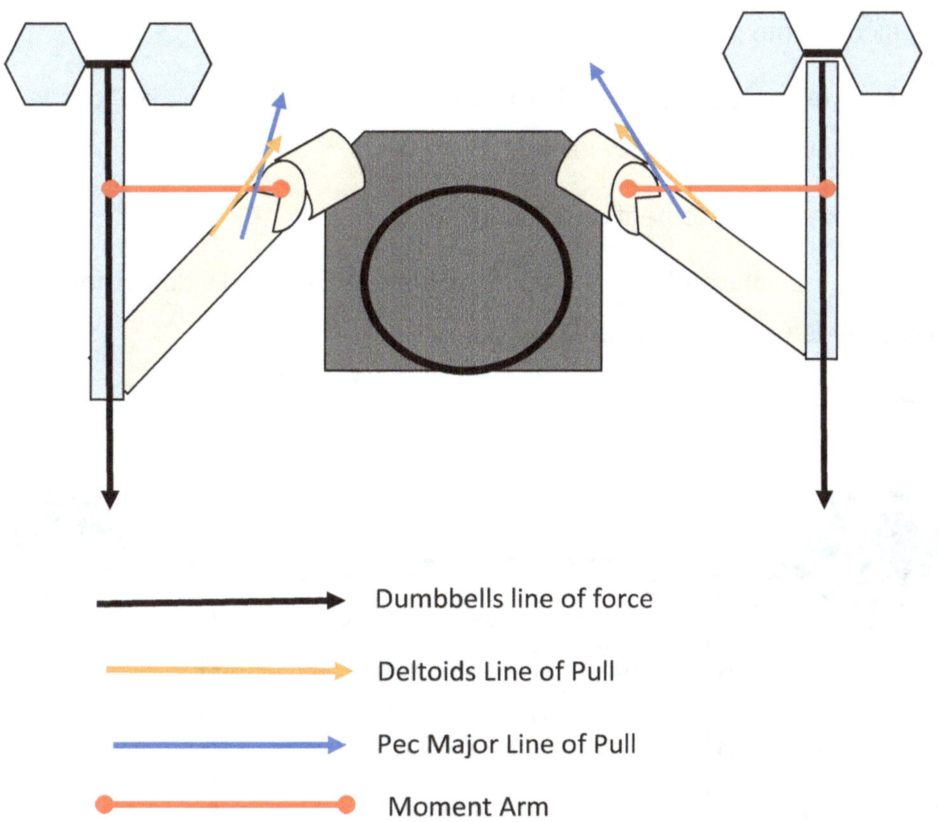

In this illustration, we have the dumbbells acting on the individual's forearm, providing an external force in the line of gravity. This force passes through the elbow joint but at a distance from the shoulder joint.

Thus, no moment arm exists between the elbows axis and the dumbbells line of force. However, a moment arm exists between the shoulder axis and the dumbbell line of force.

This means that this external force results in shoulder abduction torque, pulling the arms toward gravity. To oppose shoulder abduction torque, the Pectoralis Major (in blue) and Deltoids (in orange) must work to create a sufficient force that results in opposing shoulder adduction torque.

The ability of the pecs and delts to produce sufficient forces resulting in opposing torque production depends on multiple variables, such as

- Muscle Length
- Internal moment arm
- Line of pull on the Humerus.

Did the Triceps come into play? Nope.

The Triceps being elbow extensors, didn't have to do much in terms of "torque" production to cause a counter rotation at the elbow joint.

Simple because there is no moment arm.

Friction experienced by the individual would be between the individual's torso and the bench rested on and between the feet and the ground.

Coming to the Bench Press

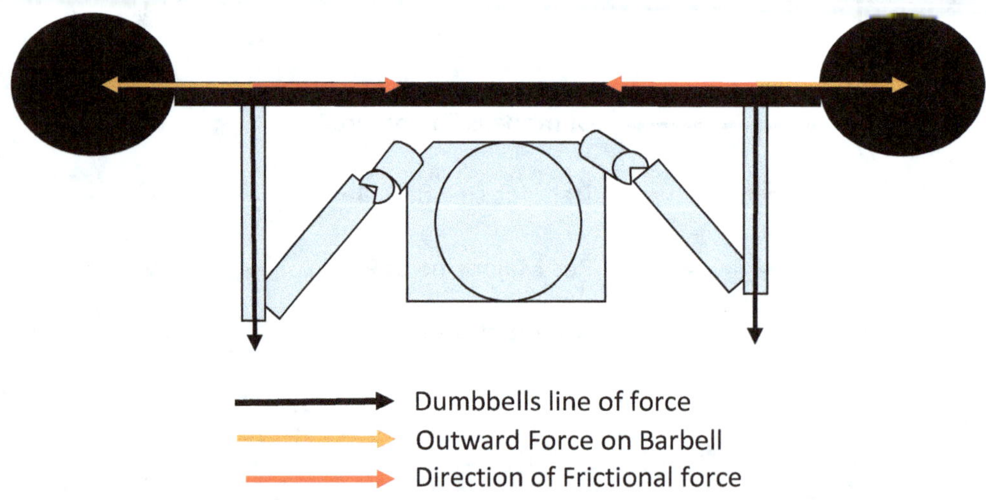

During the Bench Press, we see a similar relationship between the external forces acting on the body and the internal forces producing opposition. However, things are yet slightly different.

In the above illustration, the barbell's external forces do pass through the elbow joint and pass at a distance from the shoulder joint. This creates no moment arm between the elbows axis and the line of force but does have a moment arm between the shoulders axis and the line of force.

However, this is where frictional forces play during a bench press.

Since the barbell lies in our palms, we tend to apply force directly upwards and sideways.

In most cases, we tend to push upwards towards the right (Orange line). This creates frictional forces that prevent our hands from slipping toward the right. Hence, we have an opposing force (red line), Frictional Force.

Let's see what this hidden force offers us.

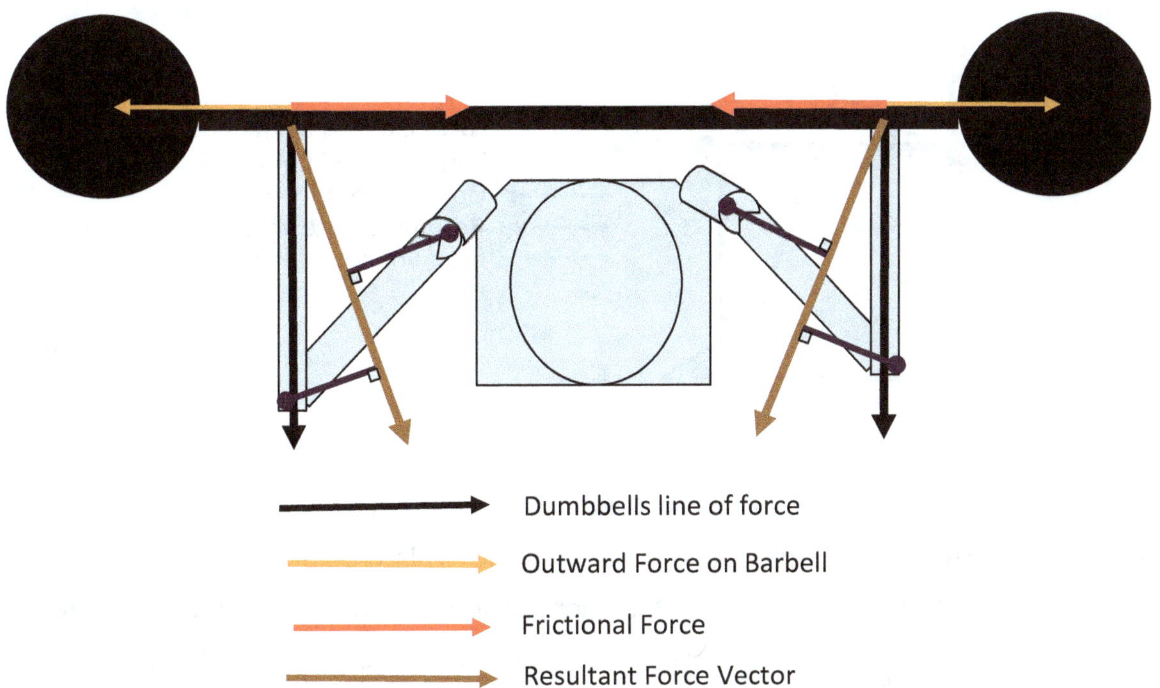

Here, we have two additional vectors (Light brown). This vector results from two forces: The downward force of the barbell and the Frictional Force opposing the outward push exerted on the barbell by the individual.

The magnitude of this resultant vector will depend on the relative magnitudes of the barbell on the forearm and the outward pushing force placed on the barbell.

This new vector now creates two-moment arms. There is a moment arm between the line of force, the elbow joint, and the shoulder joint. At the shoulder, we have shoulder abduction torque, and at the elbow, we have elbow flexion torque. Hence, the Pectoralis Major and The Deltoids must function to oppose this external torque by producing sufficient forces to create shoulder Adduction torque.

The Triceps have to function to produce sufficient forces to create elbow extension torque! Thus, the Triceps are not necessarily producing significant forces to cause rotation in the Dumbbell Press but so required to produce sufficient force during a Barbell Press. The same concept applies during a wall sit exercise.

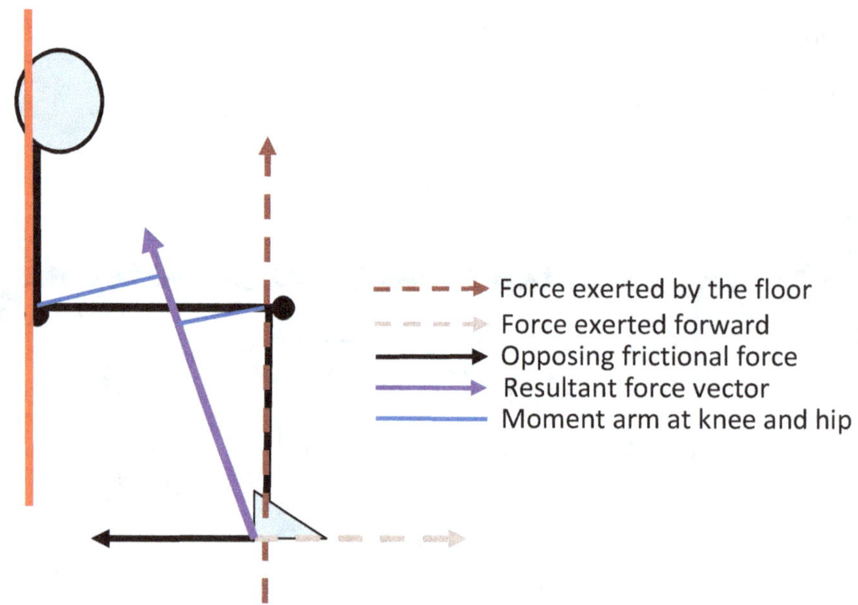

During a wall sit, we exert force into the ground, which exerts a similar magnitude right back at us through the point of force application on the ground. This creates on force vector. Friction prevents the feet from sliding forward on the floor between our feet and the ground. Hence we have a force vector that comprises frictional force. The two force vectors: the ground reaction force on feet and frictional force, creates a resultant vector angled closer to the upward ground reaction force. This vector now has some perpendicular distance between the hip and knee joints.

Thus, there exists a moment arm which creates hip flexion torque and knee flexion torque. To counter hip flexion torque, the hip extensors would have to work to create sufficient forces that result in hip extension torque. Moreover, the knee extensors would have to create sufficient forces that result in knee extension torque.

5.3 Shear Force

Forces created between the contact surfaces of two objects in contact are called Shearing Forces. However, there needs to be some linear translation/motion between the two objects, whereby the forces acting on the two objects are in opposite directions.

As seen above, shearing forces have been created between the two blocks' contact surfaces. We covered previously, how friction opposes motion between objects in contact with one another. In this case, friction plays a role in opposing shearing forces occurring at the contact surfaces of the blocks.

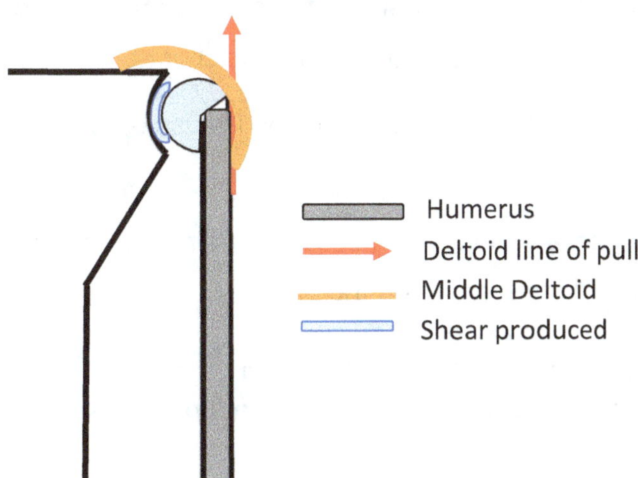

The following illustration showcases the glenohumeral joint, where the middle deltoid produces forces to abduct the upper arm against gravity.

A shearing force exists between the articulations of the glenoid fossa and the humeral head. As the deltoid begins to produce forces to abduct the upper arm, the initial outcome would result in translatory forces that work to pull on the humerus linearly. This translatory motion creates shear between the contact surfaces of the humeral head and the glenoid fossa (socket). In this example, shear would be considered a joint force.

Here friction would play a role in opposing shearing forces that take place. However, the magnitude of friction would depend upon the material that makes up the connective tissue forming the joint capsule. Since connective tissues are smooth and covered with synovial fluid, the friction experienced would be considerably less. Hence in this situation, we would rely on active and passive structures to hold the joint in place and allow smooth movement.

6. FORCE AND STRESS

Stress, in terms of biomechanics, can be defined as a constraining force or influence. Many considered stress to be considered negative, something that causes damage, sadness, or destruction. But when it comes to the human body, we must understand that stressors are all around us. Stress is forces acting on the human body, in other words, Mechanical Stress. Specifically, Mechanical Stress is the force provided over an object/tissue's cross-sectional area.

An external load on a limb stresses the area over which it acts. Moreover, we can internally produce sufficient forces to offset such stressors. Internal force production can be considered stress because it is applied to structures over which it acts.

Stress can cause adaptation, such as skeletal muscle hypertrophy, mitochondrial biogenesis, strength gains, etc.

Moreover, stress can also lead to excessive strain and injuries over time. The stress here is external and internal forces acting on the body.

The popular saying, "you either use it or lose it," basically talks about how stress is essential for certain adaptations. Stressing tissues leads to adaptive responses that otherwise may not occur without stress.

Stressors that we experience:

6.1 Tension

Forces that act on a structure to cause it to stretch. For instance, while pulling a rubber band apart, the band starts to develop tension within itself as we keep pulling. The tension produced resists the "pulling" of the band. Moreover, tension can also be considered axial stress, or stress placed longitudinally on an object.

Tension can also be considered as Tensile Stress, which tends to develop along an object/structure due to forces pulling apart the object/structure longitudinally but in opposite directions.

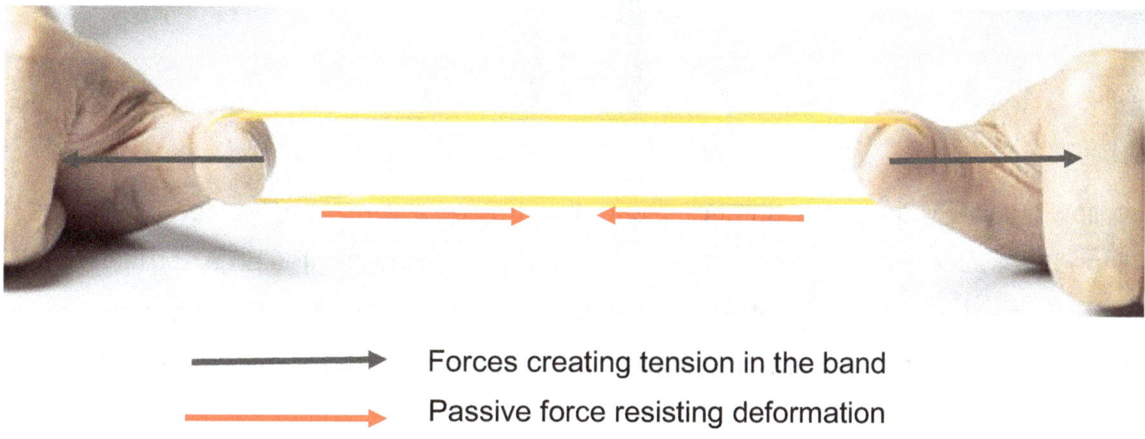

This can be visualized when talking about skeletal muscle as well.

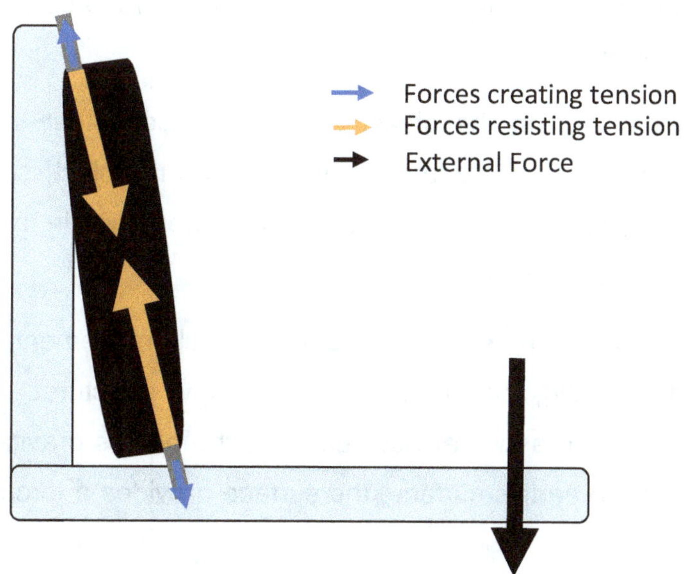

In the above example, we notice how the external load placed on the arm results in torque around the given joint. Considering this an elbow joint, we would experience elbow extension torque.

This leads to the Bicep Brachii (an elbow flexor) experiencing a stretch, which requires it to produce active forces to resist the stretch. Here, the active force is termed "Mechanical Tension."

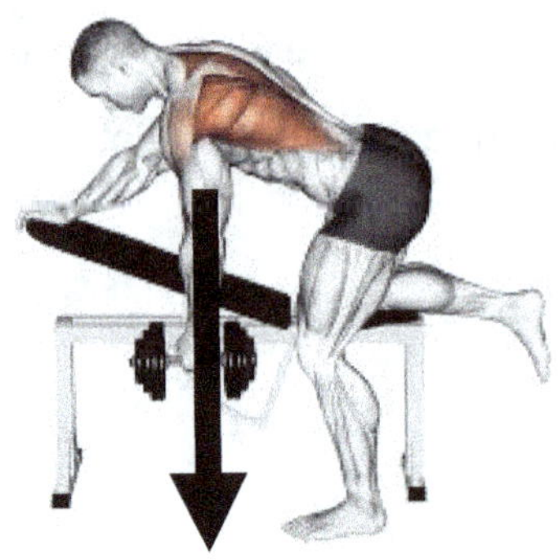

In the following illustration, the dumbbell and the trainee's arm can be considered as the external load that accelerates downwards due to gravity and thus creates an external force. This external force creates a "pulling" effect on the tissues surrounding the Glenohumeral, Elbow, and Wrist Joints. Soft tissues like ligaments and tendons are being loaded, and bones are subjected to tensile stress.

6.2 Compression

Compression is another type of axial stress created when two forces act toward each other from opposite directions on an object. Think of two forces acting on a diet coke can to flatten the can.

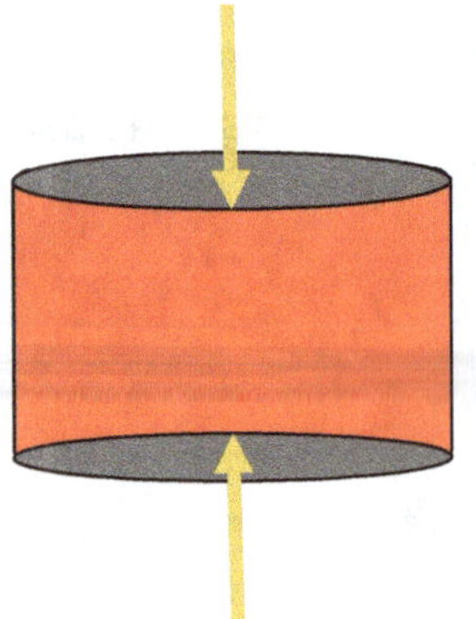

Compressive forces acting on the object are facing each other in opposite directions. Depending on the material that makes up this object, such forces could either completely compress it or just create an indentation in the direction in which the forces act on the thing.

Compressive forces act on the femoral head during daily movement, commonly including standing, walking, or squatting. Our bony structures experience compressive forces as long as we are subjected to the earth's gravitational pull. As we apply force on the earth's surface, the surface provides a force right back

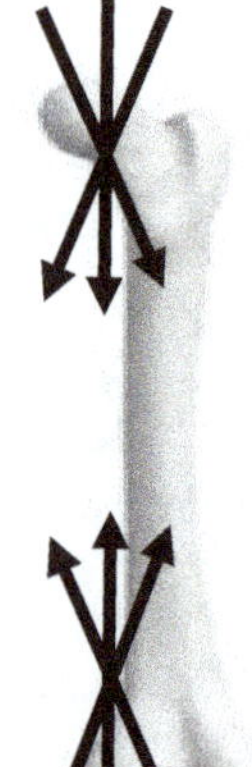

at us (reaction force). Hence we have two vectors working to create compression at various joints in the body.

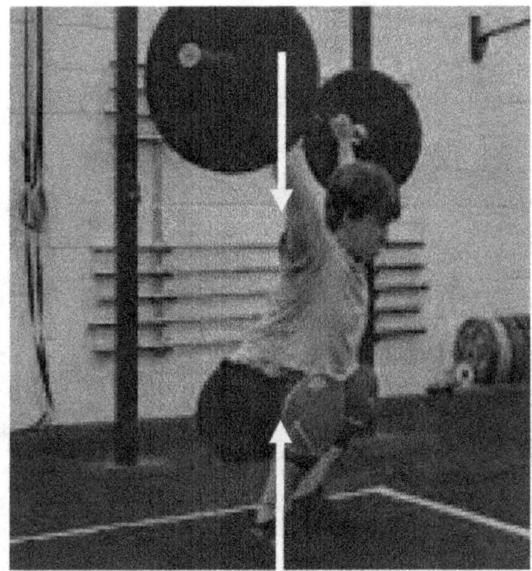

An overhead squat is considered an "axially" loaded movement due to creating axial stressors across multiple joints, specifically the individual intervertebral joints.

6.3 Shear

Another stressor that we often experience is Shear. While tensile and compressive stress act on an object longitudinally, shear affects an object transversally.

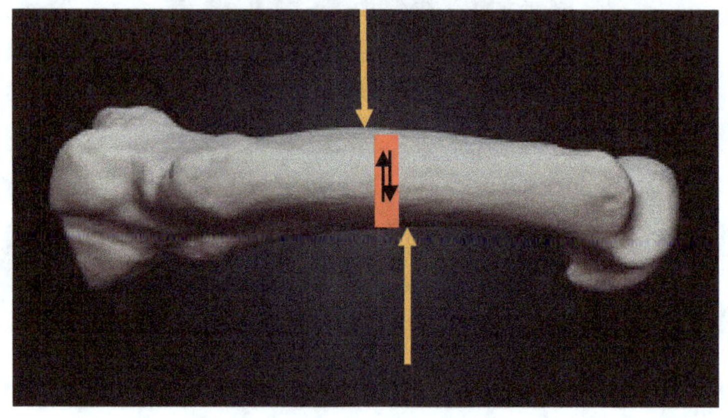

→ Forces acting externally

→ Shear forces experienced

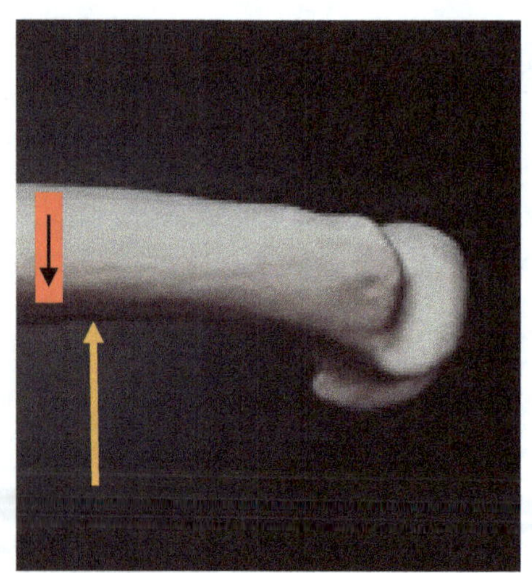

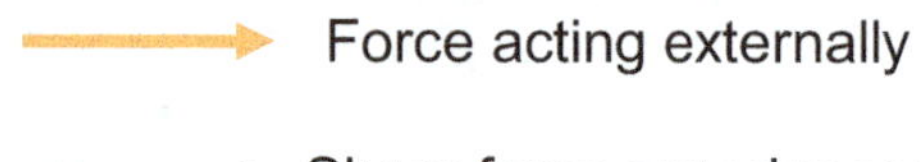

→ Force acting externally

→ Shear force experienced

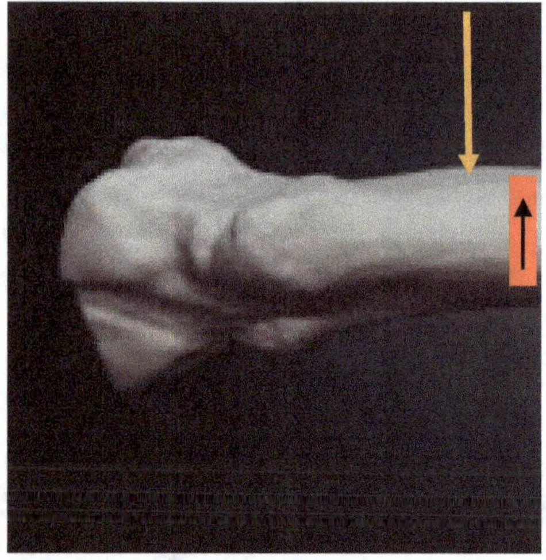

→ Force acting externally

→ Shear force experienced

In this example, there exist shear forces on bony segment. The two forces acting toward each other but opposite in direction create shear.

When analyzing each half of the bony segment, we see how to maintain constant equilibrium, there exists an force acting upwards to counter the downward force in the left half. Moreover, a downward force exists to counter the upward force in the righ half.

These two opposing forces that are created within the bony segement is Shear.

Summary of forces acting on the body, externally and internally.

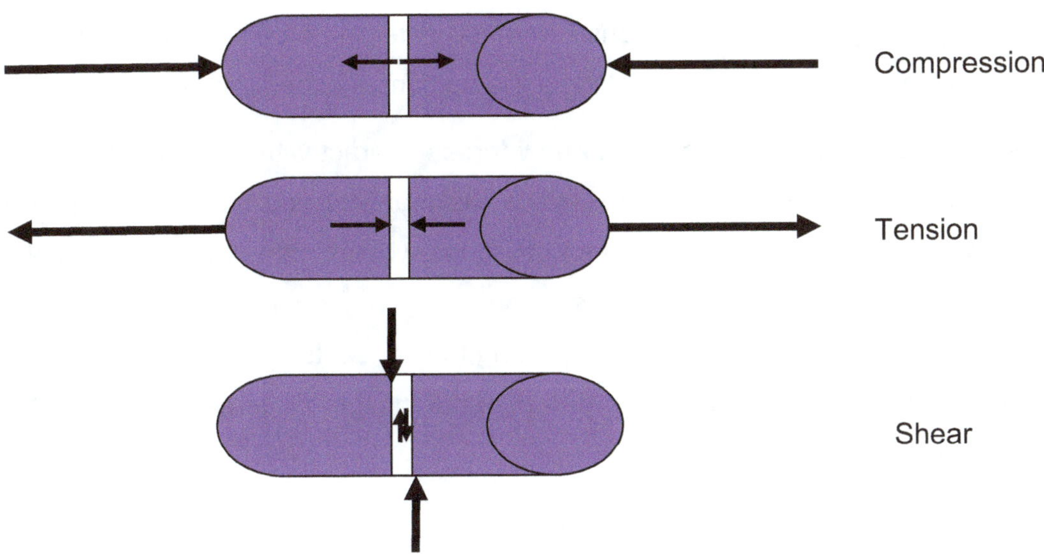

6.4 Distraction Force or Joint Distraction Force

A distraction force is a force that causes a joint to start separating from one another. Any force that leads to the separation of the articulation between two structures forming a joint.

In the following example, distraction forces will be created at the Glenohumeral Joint.

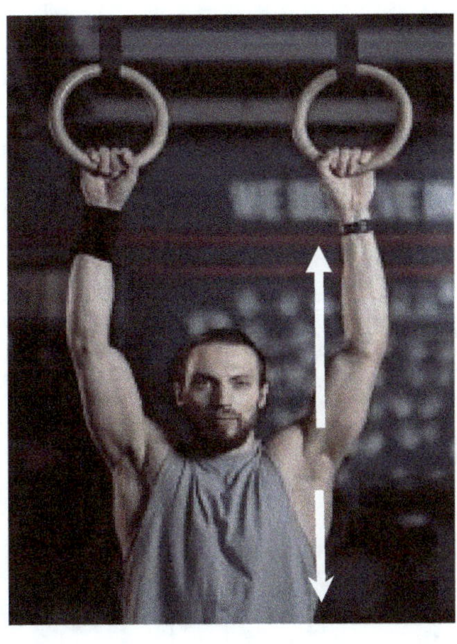

Since the individual is hanging on the rings, the rings would create a counterforce that would aim to pull on the individual. This is done to create an equilibrium.

The pull of the rings on the individual creates distraction forces at the Glenohumeral Joint.

A healthy individual has the necessary connective tissue to resist the outcome of distraction forces. Often, this is never the case unless an individual has connective tissue injuries. Connective tissues like ligaments get taut up as the rings pull on the individual. Thus, although distraction forces were created, they were checked by healthy and functioning connective tissues.

PUTTING IT ALL **TOGETHER**

Before I end my first e-book, I want to convey that humans do not experience a single external force in isolation. Moving around, lifting weights, and general exercises are an amalgamation of multiple forces interacting with us. In response to these external forces and their implications, we produce internal forces to counter or overcome the outcomes experienced.

I hope this e-book has helped you understand how forces interact with us and how we interact with forces on a day-to-day basis during exercises, as many of you sit to read this e-book. Understanding the concepts of force enhances knowledge when it comes to exercise selection, exercise progression, and exercise technique. Many may not realize this, but as exercise professionals, we must realize that exercise is applying the concepts of force to elicit a favorable adaptation down the line. Well-planned and thoughtful usage of force would elicit these adaptations.

I wish you the best, and I hope you enjoyed this book.

See you soon at the next one.

REFERENCES

1. Joint Structure and Function: A Comprehensive Analysis by Cynthia Noappliesmela Levangie (Editions 1 and 6)
2. Resistance Training Specialist by Tom Purvis (Exerciseprofessional.com)
3. Kinesiology: The Skeletal System and Muscle Function by Joseph Muscolino
4. Biomechanics of Sports and Exercise by Peter M. McGinnis (3rd Edition)
5. Biomechanics of Human Motion by Barney F. LeVeau

www.ingramcontent.com/pod-product-compliance
Lightning Source LLC
Chambersburg PA
CBHW081448250726
48662CB00009B/2999